Quick Look Nursing:

Fluids and Electrolytes

Second Edition

MARY BAUMBERGER-HENRY, DNSc, RN
Widener University
Chester, Pennsylvania

JONES AND BARTLETT PUBLISHERS
Sudbury, Massachusetts
BOSTON   TORONTO   LONDON   SINGAPORE

World Headquarters
Jones and Bartlett Publishers
40 Tall Pine Drive
Sudbury, MA 01776
978-443-5000
info@jbpub.com
www.jbpub.com

Jones and Bartlett Publishers Canada
6339 Ormindale Way
Mississauga, Ontario L5V 1J2
Canada

Jones and Bartlett Publishers
International
Barb House, Barb Mews
London W6 7PA
United Kingdom

Jones and Bartlett's books and products are available through most bookstores and online booksellers. To contact Jones and Bartlett Publishers directly, call 800-832-0034, fax 978-443-8000, or visit our website www.jbpub.com.

Substantial discounts on bulk quantities of Jones and Bartlett's publications are available to corporations, professional associations, and other qualified organizations. For details and specific discount information, contact the special sales department at Jones and Bartlett via the above contact information or send an email to specialsales@jbpub.com..

The authors, editor, and publisher have made every effort to provide accurate information. However, they are not responsible for errors, omissions, or for any outcomes related to the use of the contents of this book and take no responsibility for the use of the products and procedures described. Treatments and side effects described in this book may not be applicable to all people; likewise, some people may require a dose or experience a side effect that is not described herein. Drugs and medical devices are discussed that may have limited availability controlled by the Food and Drug Administration (FDA) for use only in a research study or clinical trial. Research, clinical practice, and government regulations often change the accepted standard in this field. When consideration is being given to use of any drug in the clinical setting, the health care provider or reader is responsible for determining FDA status of the drug, reading the package insert, and reviewing prescribing information for the most up-to-date recommendations on dose, precautions, and contraindications, and determining the appropriate usage for the product. This is especially important in the case of drugs that are new or seldom used.

Production Credits
Executive Editor: Kevin Sullivan
Acquisitions Editor: Emily Ekle
Associate Editor: Amy Sibley
Editorial Assistant: Patricia Donnelly
Production Director: Amy Rose
Production Editor: Carolyn F. Rogers
Senior Marketing Manager: Katrina Gosek
Associate Marketing Manager: Rebecca Wasley
Manufacturing and Inventory Coordinator: Amy Bacus
Compositor: Auburn Associates, Inc.
Cover Illustrator: Cara Judd
Cover Layout Artist: Timothy Dziewit
Printing and Binding: Malloy, Inc.
Cover Printing: Malloy, Inc.

Library of Congress Cataloging-in-Publication Data
Baumberger-Henry, Mary.
 Fluids and electrolytes / Mary Baumberger-Henry. — 2nd ed.
  p. ; cm. — (Quick look nursing)
 Includes bibliographical references and index.
 ISBN-13: 978-0-7637-5133-3 (pbk.)
 ISBN-10: 0-7637-5133-2 (pbk.)
 1. Water-electrolyte imbalances—Nursing. 2. Body fluid
disorders—Nursing. 3. Water-electrolyte balance (Physiology) I.
Title. II. Series.
 [DNLM: 1. Water-Electrolyte Imbalance—Nurses' Instruction. WD 220
B347f 2008]
 RC630.B28 2008
 616.3'9920231—dc22
                          2007031564
6048

Printed in the United States of America
11 10 09 08 07   10 9 8 7 6 5 4 3 2 1

DEDICATION

This book is dedicated to my husband, James Henry, and to my brother-in-law, Tomas Henry, for all of their time, patience, and humor. They helped in more ways than they know. It is also dedicated to my two daughters, Kaytlin and Brittany, for their support and encouragement from the beginning to the completion of this undertaking.

CONTENTS

vi

PREFACE

Quick Look Nursing: Fluids and Electrolytes, Second Edition is written for nursing students or students in allied health fields. It is written in a progressive style, starting with the cellular membrane; advancing to tissues, organs, and systems; and finishing with the disease processes that affect the complete system. A physiological approach to the basic concepts of fluids and electrolytes and the need for acid–base balance in the body is used. Content includes disturbances of these properties and how the imbalance may affect the various systems of the body and consequent disease states.

Each chapter features various learning tools that provide the reader with important facts. Starting at the cellular level, Part I looks at the cell's membrane and how solutes are transported in and out of the cell. Part II involves the most important electrolytes in the body and how increased or decreased levels can influence body fluids and related clinical manifestations. Acid–base balance is the main content in Part III, with a look at metabolic and respiratory control as well as interpretation of arterial blood gases. Part IV takes the reader beyond the cell with a look at organs and how four very important systems influence fluid, electrolyte, and acid–base balance. The book culminates in Part V with disease processes that stem from imbalances in the body. Written as a supplement for a text, *Quick Look Nursing: Fluids and Electrolytes* is a quick guide—from cell to system—that assists the reader in understanding a complex topic.

ABOUT THE AUTHOR

Mary Baumberger-Henry, DNSc, RN, is an associate professor at Widener University in Chester, Pennsylvania. She completed her Bachelor of Science in Nursing at Mount Marty College, Yankton, South Dakota. After 15 years of critical care nursing in medical/surgical, cardiac, and burn units, she received a Master of Science in Critical Care and a doctorate in Nursing Science from Widener University. Dr. Baumberger-Henry is now the director of the emergency/critical care master's degree program at Widener University. She resides in New Jersey with her husband, Dr. James Henry, and two daughters, Kaytlin and Brittany Henry.

I

Basics

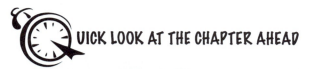

The cell is the smallest functional unit of the body. In this chapter we briefly explore the cell's function and the more important parts of its composition.

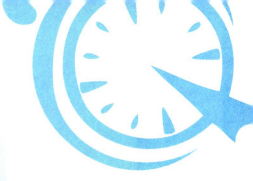

1

The Cell Membrane

TERMS

☐ Cell

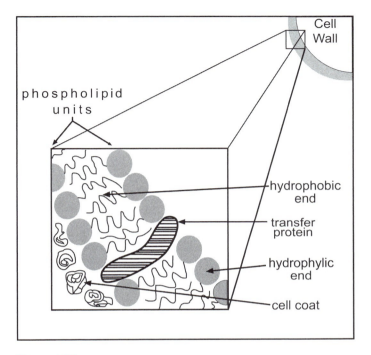

Figure 1-1 The cell membrane.

FUNCTION

The smallest autonomous functional unit of the body is the **cell.** In its fetal form it is undifferentiated, but as growth continues the cell differentiates into specific tissue types, forming organs and systems. The cell wall is a semipermeable membrane that separates the intracellular from the extracellular components, allowing for an exchange of materials through the membrane in an effort for the cell to obtain energy, synthesize complex molecules, participate in electrical events, and replicate. The cell senses signals that help it respond to changes in its environment and adapt accordingly.

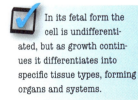

In its fetal form the cell is undifferentiated, but as growth continues it differentiates into specific tissue types, forming organs and systems.

COMPOSITION

Phospholipids

The cell wall is a semipermeable membrane that separates the intracellular from the extracellular components, allowing for an exchange of materials through the membrane in an effort for the cell to obtain energy, synthesize complex molecules, participate in electrical events, and replicate. Phospholipids are arranged with one end hydrophilic (loving water) and the other end hydrophobic (hating water). The hydrophilic head faces the outside of the membrane, retaining water and adhering to the neighboring cell. The hydrophobic tail associates with other fatty groups to exclude the hydrophilic groups. Lipid composition determines the cell membrane's degree of fluidity. At a normal temperature the composition resembles olive oil. As saturated lipids or cholesterol increases in content, the cell's membrane becomes less fluid and more stiff.

 At a normal temperature the lipid composition of the cell membrane resembles olive oil. As saturated lipids or cholesterol increases in content, the cell's membrane becomes less fluid.

Proteins

Protein molecules are the second major component of the cell membrane where most of the functions of the cellular membrane occur. They transport lipid-insoluble particles acting as carriers to pass these compounds directly through the membrane. Some proteins form ion channels for the exchange of electrolytes. The type of protein involved with a particular cell depends on that cell's function. The protein on a red blood cell has a particular flexible shape to allow the cell to thread its way through the small capillaries. In contrast, the protein of the renal tubular cell extends through the membrane to transport and exchange ions. Compounds such as glucose and nutrients are actively transported through the specific protein channels.

 Some proteins transport lipid-insoluble particles acting as carriers to pass these compounds directly through the membrane. Other proteins form ion channels for the exchange of electrolytes.

Cell Coat

Long chains of complex carbohydrates make up glycoproteins, glycolipids, and lectins that form the outside surface of the cell. This intricate coat helps in cell-to-cell recognition and adhesion. It contains antigens that label the cell as self/nonself or, as with red blood cells, contain the ABO blood group antigens. If the cell coat becomes damaged or removed, the cell does have the capability to build a new coat, but usually the cell dies.

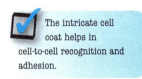

The intricate cell coat helps in cell-to-cell recognition and adhesion.

Active transport involves the use of energy to move molecules and is divided into primary and secondary active transport. Adenosine triphosphate acts as a primary source of energy that moves compounds in and out of the cells. Secondary active transport involves using the energy of a primary transport system to help carry another substance. Proteins with two binding sites help with this type of cotransportation. Primary and secondary active transport systems are further explained in this chapter.

2

Active Transport

TERMS
- [ ] **Concentration gradient**
- [ ] **Primary active transport**
- [ ] **Secondary active transport**

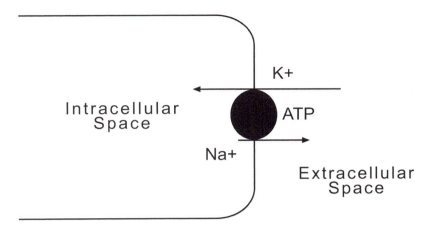

K+

Intracellular
Space

ATP

Na+

Extracellular
Space

Figure 2-1   Active transport.

The cell is constantly working, using energy and creating wastes. Mechanisms are in place for the transport of substances across the cellular membrane; some are active and others, such as osmosis, diffusion, or filtration, are passive. Active transport involves

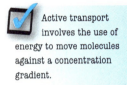

Active transport involves the use of energy to move molecules against a concentration gradient.

the use of energy to move molecules from an area of lower to an area of higher concentration and is divided into primary and secondary active transport. **Primary active transport** uses the initial source of energy to carry the substance. **Secondary active transport** harnesses the energy obtained from the primary active transport and uses it as a cotransporter of a secondary substance.

ADENOSINE TRIPHOSPHATE

Molecules too large to pass through the cell's membrane, such as glucose, require an additional source of transport. Adenosine triphosphate (ATP) is a molecule containing high-energy phosphate bonds, synthesized in the cell, that performs as a primary source of energy for moving compounds in and out of the cells. ATP helps to carry a molecule against the **concentration gradient**, the difference in concentration between an area of lesser solute concentration and an area of greater solute concentration. This energy form cannot cross the plasma membrane to be stored; therefore each cell is responsible for making its own ATP to meet its needs. Every cell has this capability, and the amount of energy needed is determined by that particular type of cell. High-energy cardiac cells require more ATP formation daily than cells with less demanding functions.

Sodium–Potassium Pump

One of the most efficient forms of active transport is the sodium–potassium pump. If sodium was allowed to accumulate inside the cell, water would follow, causing the cell to burst; therefore the sodium–potassium pump is present in all cells. This pump keeps potassium levels high and sodium levels low inside the cell and potassium levels low and sodium levels high outside the cell (Figure 2-1). The high-energy phosphate bond in ATP is split by the enzyme ATPase, releasing the energy needed to maintain the two electrolytes in their respective places against the concentration gradient. ATP is an important source of energy used by this pump to keep the vital gradient performing efficiently.

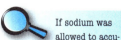 If sodium was allowed to accumulate inside the cell, water would follow, causing the cell to burst; therefore the sodium–potassium pump is present in all cells. This pump keeps potassium levels high and sodium levels low inside the cell and potassium levels low and sodium levels high outside the cell.

SECONDARY ACTIVE TRANSPORT

Secondary active transport involves using the energy of a primary transport system to help carry another substance. Proteins with two binding sites help with this type of cotransportation. Frequently, sodium occupies one of the binding sites and is accompanied by another substance, such as glucose, which is too big to pass through the cell membrane. Amino acids are another source that occupy a site and cotransport with sodium.

 Sodium, glucose, amino acids, and other substances prefer to bind with protein for cotransportation.

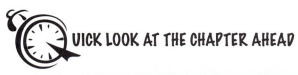

Passive transport depends on the concentration of fluids. Two examples of passive transportation are diffusion and osmosis. Both types of passive transportation and a comparison of osmolality and osmolarity are explained in this chapter.

3

Osmolality and Passive Transport

TERMS
- ☐ **Diffusion**
- ☐ **Osmolality**
- ☐ **Osmolarity**
- ☐ **Osmosis**

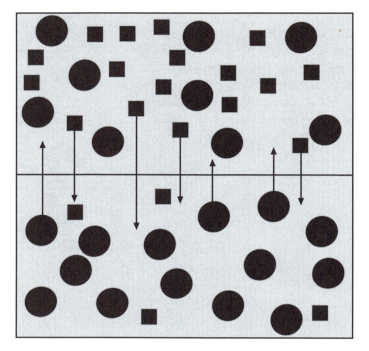

Figure 3-1 Osmolality and passive transport.

Frequently, the terms **osmolarity**, the osmolar concentration of 1 L of solution, and **osmolality**, the osmolar concentration in 1 kg of water, are used interchangeably. This switching of terms is accepted because 1 L of water is equal to 1 kg in weight. However, osmolarity is used most often when referring to solutions and fluids outside the body and osmolality when referring to fluids inside the body.

OSMOLALITY

The semipermeable membrane of the cell allows a constant movement of some solutes, whereas others remain confined within their boundaries. Whether confined or free to move, a solution's osmotic concentration is determined by the amount of dissolved particles. The normal

 The normal range for serum osmolality is 280–295 mOsm/kg. Blood values that fall below 280 mOsm/kg indicate a hypoosmolar state and those that are greater than 295 mOsm/kg are considered a hyperosmolar state.

range for serum osmolality is 275–295 mOsm/kg (milliosmols per kilogram). Blood values that fall below this range indicate a hypoosmolar state and those that are greater than 295 mOsm/kg are considered a hyperosmolar state. The following formula is used to determine serum osmolality:

$$2 \times \text{serum Na} + \frac{\text{BUN}}{3} + \frac{\text{glucose}}{18} = \text{serum osmolality (mOsm/kg)}$$

where BUN is blood urea nitrogen. However, sodium is the primary ion in the extracellular fluid (range, 136–148 mEq/L); therefore simply doubling the serum sodium level gives one an estimate of the total plasma osmolality.

PASSIVE TRANSPORT

Whether ions are extracellular, such as sodium and chloride, or are primarily intracellular, such as potassium and phosphate, the equilibrium of fluids and electrolytes is controlled through active and passive transport. Passive transport depends on the osmolarity of a solution involving movement from areas of greater to lesser concentration. A hyperosmolar solution has a higher concentration of ions as compared with a hypoosmolar solution. Osmosis and diffusion are two examples of passive transport.

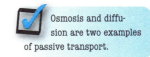
Osmosis and diffusion are two examples of passive transport.

Osmosis

Water is constantly shifting through the semipermeable membrane of the cell to the interstitial space or to the blood vessels and back in an effort to maintain a state of equilibrium. Unlike electrolytes, which require a special transport mechanism, water flows freely through the cell membrane by traveling between the intracellular and extracellular compartments using the passive movement of osmosis. **Osmosis** is the distribution of

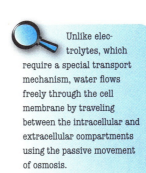
Unlike electrolytes, which require a special transport mechanism, water flows freely through the cell membrane by traveling between the intracellular and extracellular compartments using the passive movement of osmosis.

water from a lesser area of solute concentration to a higher area of solute concentration. The direction is determined by the concentration of particles on either side of the cell membrane. For example, when a state of intracellular hyperosmolarity exists, water shifts from the area of lower solute concentration with more fluid, the interstitial area, to the intracellular area with a higher solute concentration and less fluid. Osmosis stops when the concentration of solutes on both sides of the membrane becomes equalized.

Diffusion

Diffusion refers to the movement of solutes from a state of higher concentration to that of a lower concentration. Like osmosis, this is a passive movement that does not require energy. The rate of movement, however, depends on the availability of openings in the cell membrane, the total number of particles, and the kinetic movement of the particles.

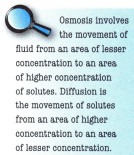

Osmosis involves the movement of fluid from an area of lesser concentration to an area of higher concentration of solutes. Diffusion is the movement of solutes from an area of higher concentration to an area of lesser concentration.

   Diffusion is affected by increased temperatures. A higher temperature increases the thermal motion of the molecules, creating a greater diffusion process. Molecules diffuse until there is an equal distribution on both sides of the membrane.

The body can be divided into two major fluid compartments, the intracellular and extracellular. The extracellular compartment is further subdivided into the interstitial, or fluid spaces between cells, and the intravascular, or blood vessel, compartments. A third fluid compartment contains the transcellular fluids of the body. Fluids are constantly shifting among the body's compartments to maintain a state of homeostasis. In this chapter we explain the percentage of body fluid in these three body compartments and which electrolytes are most abundant in each area.

4

Fluid Compartments

TERMS
- [ ] **Extracellular fluid**
- [ ] **Interstitial fluid**
- [ ] **Intracellular fluid**
- [ ] **Transcellular fluid**

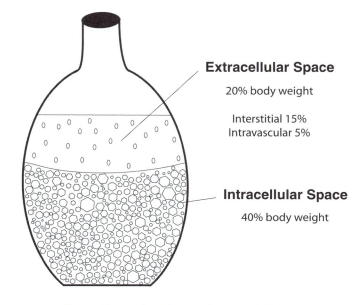

Extracellular Space

20% body weight

Interstitial 15%
Intravascular 5%

Intracellular Space

40% body weight

Total Body Fluid = 60% Body Weight

Figure 4-1 Fluid compartments.

In the healthy individual the fluid compartments maintain a constant homeostatic environment. The intake of fluids throughout the day should equal the amount that is lost. To stay within a narrow physiological range the body exchanges solutes and water between compartments, compensating for conditions that increase or decrease losses.

The body can be divided into two major fluid compartments, the intracellular, which is fluid inside the cell, and the extracellular, which is fluid outside the cell. The cell membrane serves as the initial barrier for substances to move to or from the intracellular compartment.

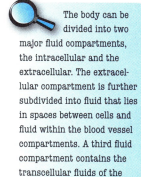

The body can be divided into two major fluid compartments, the intracellular and the extracellular. The extracellular compartment is further subdivided into fluid that lies in spaces between cells and fluid within the blood vessel compartments. A third fluid compartment contains the transcellular fluids of the body.

INTRACELLULAR FLUID

The **intracellular fluid**, or water within the billions of body cells, makes up approximately two-thirds of the body's water, or 40% of body weight. The larger of the two compartments, the intracellular fluid compartment is rich in electrolytes, potassium, magnesium, inorganic and organic phosphates, and proteins.

EXTRACELLULAR FLUID

The **extracellular fluid compartment** contains all the fluid outside the cell and is further divided into the interstitial or fluid spaces between cells and the intravascular or blood vessel compartments. The **interstitial fluid** accounts for approximately 15% of body weight, and the intravascular compartment

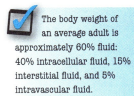 The body weight of an average adult is approximately 60% fluid: 40% intracellular fluid, 15% interstitial fluid, and 5% intravascular fluid.

contributes only 5% to the body weight of an average adult. The extracellular fluid is rich in electrolytes: sodium, chloride, and bicarbonate. When blood tests of serum electrolytes are drawn, it is the extracellular fluid that is measured for electrolyte levels, not the intracellular fluid.

TRANSCELLULAR FLUID

A third compartment is the **transcellular fluid compartment**. This compartment includes fluid located in the peritoneal, pleural, and pericardial cavities as well as cerebrospinal fluid, fluid within the joint spaces, lymph system, eyes, and gastrointestinal tract. The transcellular space contributes approximately 1% of the body fluid, and significant gains or losses do not occur on a daily basis; however, increases may occur with certain physiological conditions or traumatic events such as abdominal compartment syndrome. If there is a significant increase in fluid within

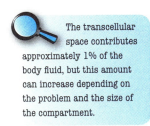 The transcellular space contributes approximately 1% of the body fluid, but this amount can increase depending on the problem and the size of the compartment.

the transcellular space, it may be termed a *third space* because the fluid is not easily exchanged with the remaining extracellular fluid.

TOTAL BODY WATER

Total body water is the equivalent of the fluids that exist in all the fluid compartments. This is approximately 60% of the body weight of an average adult. Expressed in kilograms, 1 L of fluid is the equivalent of 2.2 lb (1 kg).

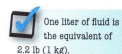

One liter of fluid is the equivalent of 2.2 lb (1 kg).

Because fat is hydrophobic fat cells contain less water; therefore an obese person has less body water than a normal-weight adult. In contrast to this, a newborn infant's weight is approximately 75–80% total body water. As we age the body's water content decreases to approximately 45% due to the loss of skeletal muscle mass.

QUICK LOOK AT THE CHAPTER AHEAD

Sodium, potassium, calcium, and magnesium are four major cations in the body. Important anions are bicarbonate, chloride, phosphate, and proteins. In this chapter we briefly explain the concentrations of these ions inside and outside the cell.

5

Cations and Anions

C A T I O N S	Extracellular	Intracellular
	Sodium 135-148mEq/L Potassium 3.5-5.3mEq/L Calcium 8.5-10.5mg/dl Magnesium 1.8-2.7mg/dl	Sodium 10-14mEq/L Potassium 140-150mEq/L Calcium <1mEq/L Magnesium 40mEq/kg
A N I O N S	Bicarbonate 23-27mEq/L Chloride 98-106mEq/L Phosphate 2.5-4.5mg/dl Proteins 16mEq/L Other anions 8mEq/L	Bicarbonate 7-10mEq/L Chloride 3-4mEq/L Phosphate 4mEq/kg Proteins 54mEq/L Other anions 31-86mEq/L

Values differ among laboratories or
by patient nutritional status

Figure 5-1 Cations and anions.

Electrolytes are divided into positively and negatively charged groups called **cation**s (+) and **anion**s (−). Single or multiple charges denote their strength, or valence. Sodium and potassium are the predominant monovalent single-charge cations, whereas chloride represents a major monovalent anion. Calcium and magnesium represent divalent double-charge cations vital in many body functions. These electrolytes are measured in milliequivalents. Divalent ions have a stronger bond than monovalent ions. For example, two monovalent anions attempt to maintain an electrochemical balance by combining with one divalent anion (e.g., $Ca^{++} + 2CL^- = CaCl_2$).

UNITY OF CHARGE

Within a single cell or the body as a whole there must be a balance of electrical charges. Every exchange between spaces must conform to this electrical unity. If a positively charged molecule moves into a cell, another positively charged molecule must leave. Likewise, all cations must be balanced with appropriate anions within a body space or within a single cell.

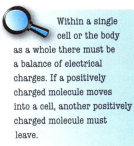

Within a single cell or the body as a whole there must be a balance of electrical charges. If a positively charged molecule moves into a cell, another positively charged molecule must leave.

ELECTROLYTE DISTRIBUTION

Electrolytes are distributed differently in the extracellular and intracellular fluid compartments. In the extracellular fluid sodium is the most abundant and powerful cation and chloride is the most abundant anion. Both sodium and chloride help maintain fluid volume in the body. Sodium is the manager of extracellular fluid osmolality. Any shift in sodium among the fluid compartments affects fluid and solute ratios.

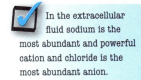

In the extracellular fluid sodium is the most abundant and powerful cation and chloride is the most abundant anion.

In the intracellular fluid compartment potassium is the most abundant cation and phosphorus the most abundant anion. As an intracellular giant, potassium helps to control the osmolality of the intracellular fluid and regulates the cell's electrical charge. If potassium is pulled from the cell, such as during acid–base imbalances, the electrical conductivity of the cell can change dramatically, resulting in a wide range of metabolic dysfunctions. Phosphorus, as the major intracellular anion, acts as a hydrogen buffer with acid–base balance. It is also vital for promoting energy storage.

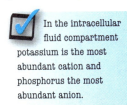

In the intracellular fluid compartment potassium is the most abundant cation and phosphorus the most abundant anion.

Other cations such as magnesium have a larger concentration in the intracellular compartment, as compared with calcium, which maintains a fairly even balance between the intracellular and extracellular compartments. Both play a major role in enzymatic processes and maintaining the electrical balance of the cell.

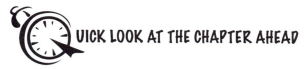

Acid–base balance must be maintained in the body fluid. This balance can easily be upset by pathological conditions such as infection, inappropriate use of medications, or trauma. At times, an acid–base imbalance can be more detrimental to the outcome of the patient's health than the initial cause of the person's illness. In this chapter we offer a brief explanation of the three regulatory mechanisms for acid–base balance in the body.

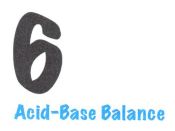

Acid-Base Balance

TERMS
☐ **Acids**

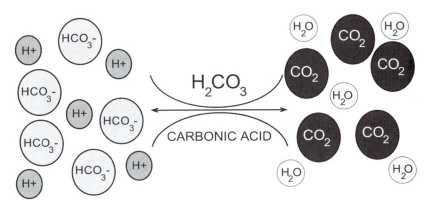

Figure 6-1 Acid–base balance.

Acid–base balance must be maintained in the body fluid. This balance can easily be upset by pathological conditions such as infection, inappropriate use of medications, or trauma—resulting in an acid–base imbalance that can be more detrimental to the outcome of the patient's health than the initial cause of the person's illness.

 At times, an acid–base imbalance can be more detrimental to the outcome of the patient's health than the initial cause of the person's illness.

The hydrogen ion (H⁺) concentration in body fluids is very small, around 0.0000001 mg/L or 10^{-7}. Because the H⁺ concentration is so low, the power of hydrogen (pH) is expressed as the negative logarithm, 10^{-7}, with the neutral point of a pH of 7.0 in the clinical setting. The pH value is inversely related to the hydrogen ion concentration; therefore as the pH decreases the solution becomes more concentrated with H⁺ and as the pH rises the solution becomes less concentrated with H⁺. In the body, fluids with a pH < 7.40 are considered to be acidic; those with a pH > 7.40 are alkaline.

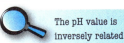 The pH value is inversely related to the hydrogen ion concentration; therefore as the pH decreases the solution becomes more concentrated with H⁺ and as the pH rises the solution becomes less concentrated with H⁺.

Acids are donors of the hydrogen ion and form as end-products of the metabolism of protein, fats, and carbohydrates. The body is constantly producing acids as end-products of metabolism. Acids must be excreted to maintain a healthy metabolic balance. A **base** substance consists of molecules that accept the hydrogen ion, helping to balance the acid content.

Three regulatory mechanisms (buffers, the respiratory system, and renal system) maintain the short- and long-term acid–base status of the body. Of the three, buffers react immediately to an acid–base imbalance by absorbing the excessive acid and preventing 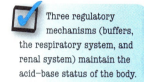 abnormal changes in the pH. The respiratory system responds in minutes to an acid imbalance but has a limited capacity and may take hours to reach maximum effectiveness. The slowest of the regulatory mechanisms is the renal system, which takes from 2 to 3 days for a maximal response but has a greater potential to maintain the proper balance for a longer period of time.

Hemoglobin and carbonic acid (H_2CO_3)– bicarbonate (HCO_3^-) are the predominant buffers in the plasma and plasma proteins. Phosphates are the primary buffers located inside the cell. Carbonic acid–bicarbonate affects both the renal and respiratory sys- 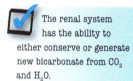 tems. The respiratory system lowers acidity by increasing the respiratory rate in an effort to exhale increased amounts of CO_2. The renal system has the ability to either conserve or generate new bicarbonate from CO_2 and H_2O (Figure 6-1).

The renal system regulates excess acid by secreting hydrogen into the urine and by reabsorbing bicarbonate in the distal tubule. CO_2 and H_2O form H_2CO_3. Carbonic anhydrase then catalyzes the reaction to form H^+ and bicarbonate (HCO_3^-). The H^+ is buffered by phosphate and ammonia and excreted while the bicarbonate is reabsorbed, helping the plasma create or maintain alkalinity (Figure 6-2).

$$CO_2 + H_2O \leftrightarrow H_2CO_3 \leftrightarrow H^+ + HCO_3^-$$

Figure 6-2 Carbonic acid–bicarbonate buffering system.

QUICK LOOK AT THE CHAPTER AHEAD

Daily fluid intake in the body should equal loss. In an effort to maintain fluid homeostasis fluids, nutrients, and waste products constantly shift among the body's cells, vasculature, and interstitial area. In this chapter we examine the different ways of fluid intake and sites of fluid loss and explain the types of pressures that influence fluid secretion and reabsorption.

7

Fluid Homeostasis

TERMS

- ☐ **Capillary hydrostatic pressure**
- ☐ **Colloidal osmotic (oncotic) pressure**

FLUID HOMEOSTASIS

Body fluid has multiple functions, including maintaining body temperature, transporting oxygen and chemicals, and eliminating wastes. Maintaining homeostasis of fluid in the various compartments of the body involves balancing intake, absorption, distribution, and excretion.

> Maintaining homeo-stasis of fluid in the various compartments of the body involves balancing intake, absorption, distribution, and excretion.

Fluid Intake

Normal fluid intake involves drinking fluids orally and ingestion through food. Other methods of fluid intake include administration of water and liquid feedings through tubes inserted into the jejunum or gastric area. Intravenous fluids can be administered to those who need additional supplements to oral intake or who are unable to ingest or

> 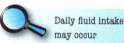 Daily fluid intake may occur naturally from
> - Drinking fluids: 1500 mL
> - Eating food: 800 mL
> - Metabolism, or oxidation of nutrients: 300 mL

absorb fluids via the gastrointestinal tract. The body also has the ability to generate its own water through metabolism or oxidation of nutrients, such as carbohydrates and fat (Figure 7-1).

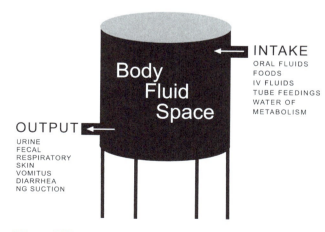

Figure 7-1   Body fluid space.

Absorption

An increased osmolality triggers the thirst center to initiate fluid intake. Once consumed, the fluid is then absorbed from the gastrointestinal tract before reaching the vascular compartment. If fluid is adminis-

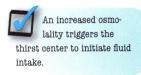

An increased osmolality triggers the thirst center to initiate fluid intake.

tered intravenously, then it is directly infused into the vascular compartment to help expand the extravascular or intravascular compartments.

Fluid Distribution Between the Plasma and Interstitial Fluid

Once fluid has been absorbed into the vascular compartment, it is distributed through capillary filtration. Only the capillaries have the ability to allow the movement of fluids and solutes through their thin walls. This is accomplished through capillary hydrostatic pressure (pushing fluid out) and colloidal osmotic (oncotic) pressure (pulling fluid in). **Capillary hydrostatic pressure** is produced by the pumping action of the heart while the **colloidal osmotic (oncotic) pressure** is the force supplied by high-molecular-weight serum proteins, such as albumin, that are too large to escape through the capillary walls.

Because these forces work against each other, the flow of fluid depends on the strongest opposing force. When capillary hydrostatic (pushing) pressure exceeds the colloidal osmotic (oncotic) pressure (pulling fluid in), movement of fluids occurs from the intravascular to the interstitial area. This movement, capillary filtration, occurs at the arterial end of the capillary. At the venous end, capillary hydrostatic pressure is less than the colloidal osmotic (oncotic) pressure; therefore fluid moves from the interstitial area into the intravascular compartment, a process known as reabsorption (Figure 7-2).

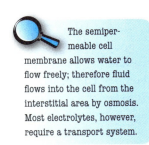

The semipermeable cell membrane allows water to flow freely; therefore fluid flows into the cell from the interstitial area by osmosis. Most electrolytes, however, require a transport system.

Fluid Excretion

The most common areas for fluid to be excreted from the body are the bowels, skin, lungs, and the renal system. Fluid is lost through the bowels in fecal matter with increased loss during bouts of diarrhea. Sweat

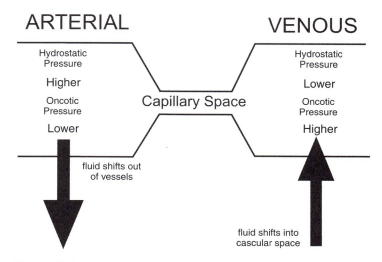

Figure 7-2   Arterial venous.

lost through skin can be either profuse or through a more natural occurrence of insensible loss. The respiratory system involves the loss of fluid through exhalation, a normal and constant event. The largest amount of fluid loss, however, occurs through urine output. The urine output of the average individual is approximately 1500 mL/day, although it can be as low as 300–500 mL/day.

Fluids can also be lost abnormally through emesis, fistulas and open weeping wounds, or hemorrhage. Tubes used for drainage of body fluids, such as nasogastric suction, are another source of fluid loss. Normally, the body compensates for such fluid losses. However, if the deficit exceeds intake, then a fluid imbalance occurs.

Daily bodily fluid loss:
- Skin: 600 mL
- Lungs: 400 mL
- Kidneys: 1500 mL
- Intestines: 100 mL

PART I • QUESTIONS

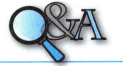

1. When a solution is more acidic, the pH value is _____, and when it has more base the pH value is _____.
   (A) Increased, decreased
   (B) Increased, increased
   (C) Decreased, increased
   (D) Decreased, decreased

2. What are the two main fluid compartments of the body?
   (A) Intracellular, extracellular
   (B) Intracellular, interstitial
   (C) Transcellular, extracellular
   (D) Intracellular, intervascular

3. What is osmosis?
   (A) Passive movement of solutes from a higher to a lower concentration.
   (B) A carrier that helps to transport glucose.
   (C) A movement activated by a thermal motion of molecules.
   (D) The movement of fluid from an area of low solute concentration to an area of higher solute concentration.

4. A simple method for estimating plasma osmolarity is to
   (A) Add the BUN and glucose
   (B) Double the serum sodium value
   (C) Subtract the fasting glucose from the serum sodium
   (D) Subtract the patient's potassium value from the serum sodium

5. Which molecule functions as a transport carrier system?
   (A) Phospholipids
   (B) Cholesterol
   (C) Carbohydrates
   (D) Protein

6. The regulatory mechanism that works the quickest in an acid–base imbalance is the
   (A) Buffering system
   (B) Renal system
   (C) Respiratory system
   (D) Sympathetic nervous system

7. An abnormal way to take in fluid would be through
   (A) Drinking fluids
   (B) Ingesting foods
   (C) Jejunostomy tube
   (D) Eating apples

8. A substance that accepts the hydrogen ion to balance the acid content is a(n)
   (A) Base
   (B) Acid
   (C) Carbonic acid
   (D) Protein

9. The most abundant cation in the extracellular fluid is
   (A) Potassium
   (B) Sodium
   (C) Chloride
   (D) Magnesium

10. The most abundant cation in the intracellular fluid is
    (A) Potassium
    (B) Sodium
    (C) Chloride
    (D) Magnesium

PART I · ANSWERS AND RATIONALES

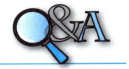

1. The correct answer is C.
   Rationale: The pH value decreases with acidic solutions and increases with alkaline solutions. Body fluids that are more acidic have a pH less than 7.40 and fluids that are alkaline have a pH greater than 7.40.

2. The correct answer is A.
   Rationale: The body is composed of two major fluid compartments, the intracellular and extracellular. The extracellular compartment is further divided into the intravascular and interstitial.

3. The correct answer is D.
   Rationale: Osmosis is the passive movement of fluid from an area of high fluid and low solute to one of low fluid and high solute. Diffusion is the passive movement of solutes and can be activated by thermal motion. Protein is a carrier that helps to transport glucose.

4. The correct answer is B.
   Rationale: Doubling the sodium value is the easiest way to evaluate a patient's serum osmolality. A more complex formula exists to determine the absolute value.

5. The correct answer is D.
   Rationale: Protein molecules help in the transport of lipids and other molecules such as glucose.

6. The correct answer is A.
   Rationale: The quickest system for correcting acid–base imbalances is the buffering system. The respiratory system is also effective but may take hours to achieve maximum benefit. The renal system may take days to achieve maximum efficiency.

7. The correct answer is C.
   Rationale: An abnormal way to take in fluids is through any type of tube or intravenous line. Normal ingestion of fluid is by mouth through the intake of fluids or food.

8. The correct answer is A.
Rationale: A base readily accepts the hydrogen ion in an attempt to correct an imbalance. Acids are donators of the hydrogen ion.

9. The correct answer is B.
Rationale: Sodium is the most abundant cation in the extracellular fluid, with a concentration of 135–145 mEq/L.

10. The correct answer is A.
Rationale: Potassium is the most abundant cation in the intracellular fluid, with a concentration of approximately 156 mEq/L.

II

Regulation of Fluids and Electrolytes

The healthy individual requires approximately 100 mL of water per 100 calories ingested to help with metabolism and the elimination of wastes. The osmolality of the body helps to determine which mechanisms will be initiated to help regulate water intake and excretion. In addition to thirst in this chapter we look at the hormones that regulate water balance: antidiuretic hormone, aldosterone, and atrial natriuretic peptide.

8

Water Balance

TERMS
☐ **Hyperosmolality**
☐ **Hypodipsia**
☐ **Osmoreceptors**

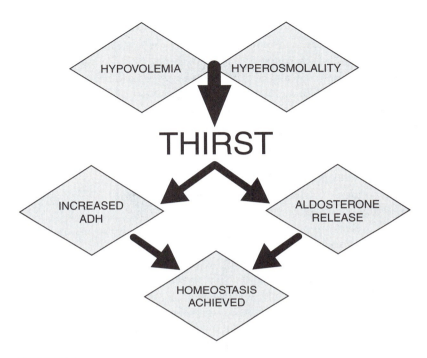

Figure 8-1 Water balance.

REGULATING WATER LEVELS

The healthy individual requires approximately 100 mL of water per 100 calories ingested to help with metabolism and the elimination of wastes. The two main body means for regulating water levels are the thirst mechanism and antidiuretic hormone (ADH). Both methods are sensitive to osmolality and to changes in extracellular fluid volume. Two hormones, aldosterone and atrial natriuretic peptide (ANP), are helpful in eliminating sodium for the regulation of fluid overload.

Thirst

Thirst occurs when a loss of body water equals or exceeds 0.5% of the total body fluid. The perception of thirst, which occurs with even

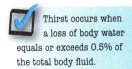
Thirst occurs when a loss of body water equals or exceeds 0.5% of the total body fluid.

the smallest loss of fluid, is one of the best regulators of water balance. **Hyperosmolality** is an event that activates the **osmoreceptors** in the hypothalamus, which trigger the sense of thirst.

Drinking fluids throughout the day is an unconscious event based on habit or social custom. One may feel thirsty when speaking for long periods of time, after consuming salty foods, or when breathing through the mouth. This dryness, however, is not truly associated with the body's hydration state. The sensation of thirst occurs when the osmoreceptors located near the thirst center of the hypothalamus are stimulated. This stimulation occurs due to cellular dehydration secondary to an increased extracellular osmolality or loss of blood. As one ages the ability to sense thirst declines, a condition known as **hypodipsia**. This condition is particularly associated with those who have suffered a stroke and places them at an increased risk for hyperosmolality and dehydration.

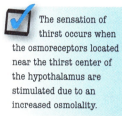 The sensation of thirst occurs when the osmoreceptors located near the thirst center of the hypothalamus are stimulated due to an increased osmolality.

The ability to sense thirst declines with age; in particular, those who have suffered a stroke are placed at an increased risk for hyperosmolality and dehydration.

Question: If my patient cannot speak because of a stroke, how can I manage one's fluid balance?

Answer: Fluid balance can be monitored through careful observation and recording of the patient's intake and output.

Antidiuretic Hormone

ADH, also known as vasopressin, is secreted by the posterior pituitary gland in response to stimulation from the hypothalamus when fluid osmolality increases secondary to a loss of water or excess sodium (hypernatremia).

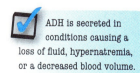 ADH is secreted in conditions causing a loss of fluid, hypernatremia, or a decreased blood volume.

ADH is also secreted if the blood pressure decreases because of decreased blood volume. Fluid is pulled from the intracellular and interstitial areas into the intravascular compartment in an effort to increase the blood pressure. This decrease in fluid in the intracellular and interstitial compartments then stimulates the hypothalamic osmoreceptors to stimulate the thirst center.

The kidneys also play a fundamental role in fluid balance. When the thirst center is stimulated, ADH is released by the posterior pituitary to act on the distal and collecting tubules of the nephron, causing reabsorption of water into the plasma. Less water is excreted into the urine. As a result, urine concentration increases and the plasma osmolality decreases and returns to normal (Figure 8-2).

The baroreceptors, located in the aorta, carotid arches, and pulmonary artery, along with receptors found in the thoracic vessels and atria are also sensitive to volume changes. When dehydration secondary to vomiting, diarrhea, or situations of excessive sweating occur these receptors sense the low fluid volume, which triggers the release of ADH.

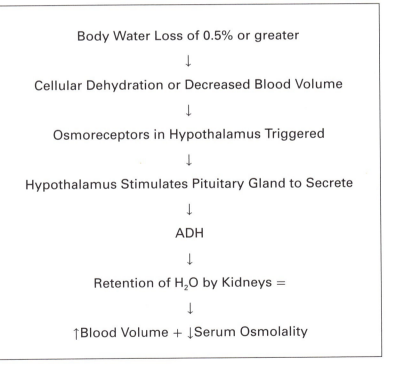

Body Water Loss of 0.5% or greater

↓

Cellular Dehydration or Decreased Blood Volume

↓

Osmoreceptors in Hypothalamus Triggered

↓

Hypothalamus Stimulates Pituitary Gland to Secrete

↓

ADH

↓

Retention of H_2O by Kidneys =

↓

↑Blood Volume + ↓Serum Osmolality

Figure 8-2 Antidiuretic hormone release and effect.

Aldosterone

Aldosterone, a mineralocorticoid, regulates
sodium balance. The secretion of aldosterone is controlled by low blood volume. In
addition, it is secreted by the adrenal cortex
when sodium levels are low and potassium

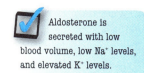

Aldosterone is
secreted with low
blood volume, low Na$^+$ levels,
and elevated K$^+$ levels.

levels are elevated. Acting on the distal tubule of the kidney, aldosterone
increases the reabsorption of sodium and excretion of potassium in the
urine. Through the reabsorption of sodium, water is drawn back into the
vascular system and fluid balance retained.

Atrial Natriuretic Peptide

ANP is a hormone released when the atria of the heart muscle are overly
stretched. Sensing this fluid overload, ANP stimulates the renal system to
vasodilate the efferent and afferent arterioles, helping to increase blood
flow to the nephron and therefore to increase the glomerular filtration
rate. Under the influence of ANP, aldosterone secretion is repressed and
the distal and collecting tubules are inhibited from reabsorbing sodium.
ADH secretion is also controlled, thus preventing retention of water via
the kidneys.

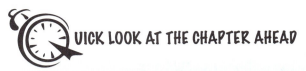

QUICK LOOK AT THE CHAPTER AHEAD

Fluid overload can occur in either the extracellular or intracellular compartments of the body. Extracellular fluid overload occurs in either the intravascular compartment or in the interstitial area. Intracellular fluid overload occurs inside the cell and is known as water intoxication. When sodium and water remain in equal proportions with each other, a situation known as isotonic fluid volume excess occurs. Excess sodium and fluid are the primary causes of extracellular overload. In this chapter we highlight the causes, manifestations, and treatment for extracellular and intracellular fluid overload.

9

Fluid Overload

TERMS
- ☐ Anasarca
- ☐ Hypervolemia
- ☐ Isotonic fluid volume excess

EXCESS INTAKE	INADEQUATE OUTPUT
EXCESS IV FLUID	CHF
BLOOD/PLASMA USE	CIRRHOSIS
HYPERTONIC FLUIDS	NEPHROTIC SYNDROME
EXCESS DIETARY SODIUM	HYPERALDOSTERONISM
COLLOID USE	LOW DIETARY PROTIEN
WATER INTOXICATION	STEROID USE
REMOBILIZATION OF EDEMA	

Figure 9-1 Excess intake and adequate output.

EXTRACELLULAR FLUID OVERLOAD

Edema is the common term associated with fluid overload found in the interstitial or lung tissue. When an overabundance of fluid occurs in the intravascular compartment, the condition is known as **hypervolemia**. The cause for overhydration may be associated with excess sodium.

Situations exist, however, when sodium and water remain in equal proportions with each other. This type of fluid overload, known as **isotonic fluid volume excess**, results from a decreased elimination of sodium and water. Normally, the body compensates and attempts to restore the fluid balance through the homeostatic mechanisms associated with antidiuretic hormone, atrial natriuretic peptide, or aldosterone. If these mechanisms malfunction due to diseases or failing organs, hypervolemia develops. The extra volume of fluid puts an excessive strain on the left side of the heart, which over time causes the heart to fail, allowing blood to back up into the pulmonary system and causing pulmonary edema. In other areas of the body dependent edema appears first in the sacrum and lower extremities and then becomes generalized throughout the body, a condition known as **anasarca** (Table 9-1).

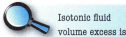 Isotonic fluid volume excess is a type of fluid overload that results from a decreased elimination of sodium and water. Sodium and water remain in equal proportions with each other.

Causes of Extracellular Fluid Overload

Fluid overload may result from excessive sodium intake through diet or administration of hypertonic fluids. Inadequate sodium or water elimination resulting in fluid overload may occur with conditions of hyperaldosteronism, Cushing's syndrome, and renal, liver, or congestive heart failure (Table 9-2). A water deficit resulting from excessive diarrhea or diaphoresis, diabetes insipidus (decreased antidiuretic hormone), may also result in a fluid imbalance.

 Fluid overload may result from excessive sodium intake through diet or administration of hypertonic fluids.

Table 9-1 Manifestations Related to Extracellular Fluid Overload

Pitting peripheral edema	Anasarca
Periorbital edema	Rapid weight gain
Shortness of breath	Moist crackles
Shift of interstitial fluid to plasma	Tachycardia
Bounding pulse and jugular venous distension	Hypertension

Table 9-2 Causes of Extracellular Fluid Overload

Increased dietary sodium intake	Diabetes insipidus
Hypertonic intravenous administration	Congestive heart failure
$D_5.45$ normal saline solution	Cirrhosis
$D_5.9$ normal saline solution	Renal failure
10% Dextrose	Cushing's syndrome
3% normal saline solution	Hyperaldosteronism

Treatment of Extracellular Fluid Overload

Excess sodium and fluid are the primary causes of extracellular overload; therefore, restricting both of them is part of the treatment. Depending on other factors, additional methods of therapy might be used. If pulmonary edema is the problem, then measures to decrease it should also be implemented. In this case maintaining a high Fowler's position with oxygen administration is necessary, along with the use of loop diuretics and morphine sulfate. If congestive heart failure is the problem, diuretics, digoxin and other inotropic and cardiovascular drugs, a low-sodium diet, and fluid restriction are the methods of treatment. Therefore one must look at the overall picture to determine which treatment is most effective.

> Excess sodium and fluid are the primary causes of extracellular overload; therefore restricting both of them is part of the treatment. However, one must look at the specific condition and overall picture to determine which treatment will be most effective.

Question: What measures should be implemented for pulmonary edema?

Answer: Keep the patient in a high Fowler's position and administer oxygen. Monitor the oxygen saturation closely as well as intake and output, especially when loop diuretics are administered.

Question: If my patient has congestive heart failure should fluids be restricted?

Answer: Yes, close monitoring of intake and output is expected along with administration of diuretics and a low-sodium diet. Along with the administration of cardiac medications, electrolytes should be carefully monitored.

INTRACELLULAR FLUID OVERLOAD

Intracellular fluid overload is known as water intoxication. Hypotonic fluid from the intravascular space moves by osmosis to an area of higher solute concentration inside the cell. Cells run the risk of rupturing if they become too overloaded with fluid; the cerebral cells are the most sensitive and first to react to excess fluid. One of the first signs of cerebral edema is head- ache, which may or may not be accompanied by irritability, confusion, or anxiety. Other

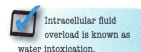
Intracellular fluid overload is known as water intoxication.

symptoms experienced may include nausea and vomiting, thirst, muscle weakness or twitching, or dyspnea on exertion (Table 9-3). If the condition is allowed to persist, a patient with water intoxication will demonstrate an elevated blood pressure, decreased pulse rate, and increased respirations.

Cells run the risk of rupturing if they become too overloaded with fluid; the cerebral cells are the most sensitive and first to react to excess fluid.

Causes of Intracellular Fluid Overload

Intracellular fluid overload results from an increased intake of intrave- nous hypotonic solutions, such as 0.45% normal saline solution and dex- trose in water (Table 9-4). Dextrose in water, which is considered to be an isotonic solution, becomes hypotonic as the body rapidly absorbs the sugar content of the solution. Another means of developing intracellu- lar fluid overload is through the electrolyte-rich gastrointestinal tract. When too much water is ingested or instilled into the gastrointestinal tract, electrolytes are lost. This may occur, for example, when excessive free water is administered through nasogastric and feeding tubes or with

Table 9-3 Manifestations of Intracellular Fluid Overload

Neurological	Gastrointestinal
Cerebral edema	Nausea and vomiting
Headache	Increased thirst
Irritability	
Confusion	Cardiac
Anxiety	Elevated blood pressure
Muscle weakness	Decreased pulse
Twitching	
Respiratory	
Dyspnea on exertion	
Increased respirations	

Table 9-4 Causes of Intracellular Fluid Overload

Hypotonic intravenous administration
0.45% normal saline solution
5% Dextrose in water*
Excessive nasogastric tube irrigation with free water
Excessive administration of free water via enteral tube feedings
Syndrome of inappropriate antidiuretic hormone
Psychogenic polydipsia

*5% Dextrose in water is considered isotonic until administered into the body where the sugar is metabolized and the solution becomes free water and, therefore, hypotonic.

excessive ingestion of water from a compulsive condition known as psychogenic polydipsia. Intracellular fluid overload may also result from renal dysfunction resulting in a decreased excretion of water or excess antidiuretic hormone secretion known as the syndrome of inappropriate antidiuretic hormone. This syndrome results in a large amount of water reabsorption by the kidneys.

 When excessive free water is administered through nasogastric and feeding tubes, water intoxication and a loss of electrolytes may occur.

Treatment of Intracellular Fluid Overload

Treatment for intracellular fluid overload is restriction of oral, enteral, and parenteral fluid intake until the serum sodium level returns to a normal value. In severe cases a hypertonic solution of 3% normal saline may be used to help shift the water overload from the cell. Caution should be used with this highly hypertonic solution. It should always be placed on an intravenous pump or controller and administered at a slow rate so the body can compensate. Also, the potential for fluid to merely shift from one compartment to another may occur, causing extracellular fluid overload. In this situation an osmotic diuretic should be added to the treatment.

Caution should be used with the use of 3% normal saline, a highly hypertonic solution. It should always be placed on an intravenous pump or controller and administered at a slow rate so the body can compensate.

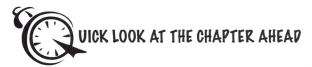

When serum sodium levels rise in the vascular system due to a fluid loss, osmosis causes water molecules to shift from the cell into the blood vessel to maintain homeostasis. Normally, this restores the fluid volume. When less fluid is available to exchange among the compartments of the body, however, the circulating blood volume decreases, causing hypovolemia and hypotension. Here we look at fluid volume deficit, the causes, and how the manifestations can start as thirst and end in hypovolemic shock.

10

Fluid Deficit

TERMS
- ☐ Hyperosmolar fluid volume deficit
- ☐ Isoosmolar fluid volume

INADEQUATE REPLACEMENT	EXCESSIVE LOSSES

POOR ORAL INTAKE
  CVA
  DEMENTIA
  NEGLECT
 	
INADEQUATE IV FLUIDS
  POOR IV ACCESS
	GI LOSSES
	  VOMITING
	  DIARRHEA
	  NG SUCTION
	RENAL
	  NEPHROSIS
	  POSTOBSTRUCTIVE
	METABOLIC
	  DIABETES MELLITUS
	  DIABETES INSIPIDUS
	SKIN
	  BURNS
	  OPEN WOUNDS
	THIRD SPACES
	  ASCITES
	  EFFUSIONS

Figure 10-1 Inadequate fluid replacement and excessive fluid losses and causes of fluid volume deficit.

DEHYDRATION
70 KG ADULT EXAMPLE

DEHYDRATION=1-3%   1-2 LITER DEFICIT
  NO CLINICAL SIGNS
  THIRST AS ONLY SYMPTOM

MODERATE DEHYDRATION=3-6% 2-4 LITER DEFICIT
  DRY MEMBRANES, POOR SKIN TURGOR,
  POSTURAL HYPOTENSION, OLIGURIA, MILD
  TACHYPNEA/TACHYCARDIA,
  HEMOCONCENTRATION

SEVERE DEHYDRATION=6-9%   4-7 LITER DEFICIT
  INCREASING SEVERITY OF ABOVE SIGNS
  HYPOTENSION WITH SHOCK, ANURIA,
  ALTERED MENTAL STATUS, ACIDOSIS

Figure 10-2 Dehydration: 70 kg adult example.

Fluid volume deficit is a total body water deficit that is associated with a loss of sodium accompanied by water. **Isoosmolar fluid volume deficit** occurs when sodium and water are lost in equal amounts. **Hyperosmolar fluid volume deficit** occurs when more fluid is lost than sodium, resulting in a higher serum osmolality than normal (> 295 mOsm/kg). Fluid volume deficit results in conditions known as dehydration and hypovolemia.

DEHYDRATION AND HYPOVOLEMIA

When serum sodium levels rise in the vascular system due to a fluid loss, osmosis causes water molecules to shift from the cell into the blood vessel to maintain homeostasis. Normally, this restores the fluid volume. The problem occurs when fluid continues to shift from the cell, causing the cell to shrink or dehydrate. With less fluid available to exchange among the compartments of the body, the circulating blood volume is decreased, causing hypovolemia and hypotension. Patients may manifest signs and symptoms of an altered level of consciousness. This can progress to a form of shock, known as hypovolemic shock, if the condition goes untreated and fluid is not replaced.

When less fluid is available to exchange among the compartments of the body, the circulating blood volume decreases, causing hypovolemia and hypotension. This can progress to hypovolemic shock if the condition goes untreated and fluid is not replaced.

CAUSES OF FLUID VOLUME DEFICIT

In addition to an inadequate fluid intake, multiple causes can result in dehydration or hypovolemia. Prolonged vomiting or diarrhea, gastrointestinal fistula, suctioning, or abscess can result in a loss of electrolytes or fluid. Metabolic problems such as diabetes insipidus contribute to an interference of synthesis, transport, or release of antidiuretic hormone (see Chapter 9), resulting in excessive diuresis. The patient produces large amounts of dilute urine and is very thirsty, but a balance between intake and output cannot occur.

Burns cause fluid to shift from the vascular to the interstitial tissues surrounding the burned area, resulting in hypovolemia. In severe cases fluid is allowed to shift to the peritoneal space along with protein and electrolytes, causing a third-spacing fluid shift known as ascites and contributing to a decrease in the circulating volume. Fever and excessive sweating allow for an increased loss of sodium and water through the skin and respiratory system.

Question: How can I tell if my patient is dehydrated?

Answer: A dehydrated patient may manifest only thirst, whereas more moderate conditions manifest dry mucous membranes, postural hypotension, and tachycardia. See Figure 10-1 for a complete list.

TREATMENT OF FLUID VOLUME DEFICIT

Clinical management depends on the cause of the condition but generally includes replacement of fluids based on the percentage of lost body weight along with treatment of the underlying problem. For example, fluid management of the burn patient is based on body weight and percentage of the burned area. Normal saline solution or lactated Ringer's solution are isotonic fluids given intravenously to expand the circulating volume. Solutions such as 5% dextrose in water are not given as replacement fluid because the glucose is immediately absorbed by the body, resulting in the administration of a hypotonic solution.

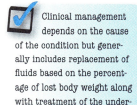

Clinical management depends on the cause of the condition but generally includes replacement of fluids based on the percentage of lost body weight along with treatment of the underlying problem.

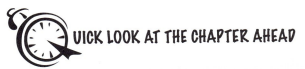

QUICK LOOK AT THE CHAPTER AHEAD

Sodium is considered the most important cation in the extracellular fluid, with a primary focus to control serum osmolality levels and water retention. Normal sodium levels in the extracellular compartment are 135–148 mEq/L and inside the cell, 10–14 mEq/L. The functions of sodium, how it is regulated, and maintaining sodium balance in the body are described in this chapter.

11

Sodium

TERMS
☐ Sodium

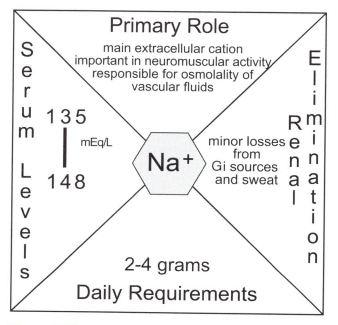

Figure 11-1 Primary role of sodium.

FUNCTIONS

Sodium is considered the most important cation in the extracellular fluid. Normal sodium levels in the extracellular compartment are 135–148 mEq/L, compared with 10–14 mEq/L inside the cell. Sodium has several different functions. Primarily, it is responsible for the osmolality of the body's vascular fluids. Doubling the serum sodium gives one a rough estimate of the body's osmolality (see Chapter 3). It also has an affinity for chloride and helps maintain acid–base balance when combined with HCO_3.

The cellular membrane is impermeable to sodium, making the electrolyte dependent on the sodium–potassium pump for transportation in and out of the cell (see Chapter 2). Sodium is known for its ability to assist with the conduction of impulses with muscle and nerve fibers, and this is accomplished via the sodium–potassium pump. As sodium shifts into the cell potassium shifts out, resulting in depolarization of the cell membrane. When sodium shifts back out of the cell potassium shifts into the cell, and the cell is considered to be repolarized. The sodium–potassium pump not only assists in maintaining fluid balance, it also assists in maintaining neuro-muscular activity. Sodium plays a major role in maintaining homeostasis within the body. When serum sodium levels become elevated or fall below normal values, problems with fluid and acid–base balance as well as impulse conduction may occur.

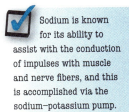 Sodium is known for its ability to assist with the conduction of impulses with muscle and nerve fibers, and this is accomplished via the sodium–potassium pump.

REGULATION OF SODIUM

Regulated by the kidneys and the hormone aldosterone, sodium's primary focus is control of serum osmolality levels and water retention. Its ability to attract fluid helps primarily with extracellular fluid distribution and control of vascular volume, which is highly important for tissue perfusion. When the vascular volume decreases, the kidney retains sodium in an effort to conserve fluid and therefore increase blood volume. The opposite occurs when the blood volume is increased (i.e., the kidney excretes sodium and water follows).

The sympathetic nervous system is responsible for the renal system's balance of sodium. The sympathetic nervous system modifies the glomerular filtration rate (GFR) within the kidneys' nephrons in response to an increase or decrease in vascular volume. The higher the GFR, the more sodium is excreted from the blood; when the GFR is decreased, more sodium is reabsorbed.

The renin-angiotensin-aldosterone mechanism also influences the amount of sodium that is secreted for maintenance of vascular volume and blood pressure (Figure 11-2). Renin is a small protein enzyme, produced by the kidney and released in response to a decreased renal blood flow. Renin then converts angiotensinogen, a circulating plasma protein, to angiotensin I. In turn, angiotensin I is converted to angiotensin II in the lungs, which initiates sodium reabsorption by the kidneys' tubules, and water follows to increase volume.

Aldosterone, a hormone secreted by the adrenal cortex, functions as part of a feedback loop that helps to conserve sodium. It acts on the renal

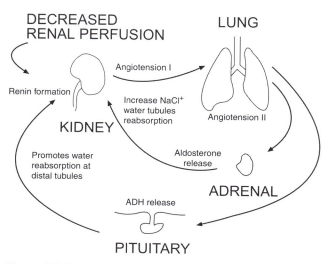

RENIN-ANGIOTENSIN-ALDOSTERONE MECHANISM

Figure 11-2 Renin-angiotensin-aldosterone mechanism.

tubules, stimulating them to hold on to water and sodium to normalize the sodium concentration and maintain fluid balance.

MAINTAINING SODIUM BALANCE

The balance of sodium within the body can be maintained through a normal dietary intake of 2 to 4 g. One teaspoon of salt is the equivalent of 2.3 g of sodium; therefore it is easy to see how supplements added to one's diet help in exceeding the normal intake to as much as 6 to 12 g/day. In addition to obvious sources

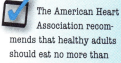

The American Heart Association recommends that healthy adults should eat no more than 2,300 mg (one teaspoon) of sodium chloride (salt) a day.

of sodium such as table salt and salty snack foods, hidden sources of sodium can quickly make up the normal daily intake (Table 11-1). When dietary sodium is increased, however, the balance is not upset in the healthy person because the kidney responds by excreting the excess intake.

Table 11-1 Dietary Sources of Sodium

Cheese	Canned soups
Seafood	Canned vegetables
Processed meats and foods	Salt
Ketchup	Snack foods containing salt

Most sodium is lost through the kidney. Sodium can also be lost through the gastrointestinal tract. Conditions that increase the loss of sodium through the gastrointestinal tract, however, must be excessive, such as prolonged vomiting and diarrhea, continuous gastrointestinal suction, frequent tap water enemas, or the flushing of gastrointestinal tubes with distilled water. Extensive burns can also result in the loss of sodium through the skin. Sweating may contribute to sodium loss through the skin; however, the loss is usually minimal unless a condition of excessive sweating exists, such as through strenuous and prolonged exercise.

Question: What should I tell my patients who want to reduce sodium in their diet?

Answer:

- Choose fresh or frozen food items.
- If using canned foods, observe the label closely.
- For snacks select unsalted nuts, seeds, crackers, fruit, or fresh vegetables.
- Select unsalted fat-free broths and bouillons and use dried beans, peas, or lentils instead of canned vegetables when making soups or homemade dishes.
- Use dairy products (i.e., milk, cheese, yogurt) that are fat free or low fat and low sodium.
- Ask for your dish to be prepared without salt when dining out.
- Do not add salt; instead, use spices, herbs, or lemon juice to enhance the taste of food.

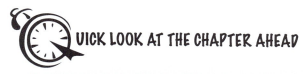

QUICK LOOK AT THE CHAPTER AHEAD

Hypernatremia occurs when the serum sodium level exceeds 148 mEq/L. An elevated serum sodium level may be caused by either a greater loss of water compared with salt or an acute gain of salt compared with water. In this chapter we describe the conditions that may cause an excessive water loss or sodium intake, along with the manifestations of hypernatremia and treatment.

12

Hypernatremia

TERMS
☐ **Hypernatremia**

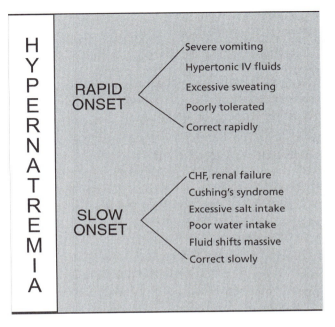

Figure 12-1 Rapid onset, slow onset.

CAUSES

Hypernatremia occurs when the serum sodium level exceeds 148 mEq/L. The osmolality in hypernatremia generally exceeds 295 mOsm/kg because it is an imbalance between the sodium and water levels in the body. Hypernatremia may be caused by either a greater loss of water compared with salt or an acute gain of salt compared with water. Table 12-1 lists examples of theses causes. If sodium levels are increased, water flows via osmosis from inside and around the cell into the intravascular compartment. This results in intracellular and interstitial dehydration and may potentially lead to hypervolemia as fluid flows into the intravascular space.

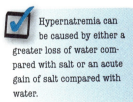

Hypernatremia can be caused by either a greater loss of water compared with salt or an acute gain of salt compared with water.

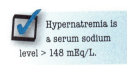

Hypernatremia is a serum sodium level > 148 mEq/L.

Table 12-1 Causes of Hypernatremia

Water Loss	Excessive Sodium Intake
Diabetes insipidus	Hypertonic intravenous solutions
Watery diarrhea	$D_5$1/2NSS
Hypertonic tube feedings	D_5LR
Hyperventilation	D_5 NSS
Excessive sweating	3% NSS
Inability to drink water (e.g.,	Total parenteral nutrition
unconscious patient	Corticosteroids
or confused elderly)	

Water Loss

A variety of situations exists that may result in an excessive loss of water from the body. Water may be lost from the body via urine as with diabetes insipidus (see Chapter 43) or with shifts between the intracellular fluid and extracellular fluid compartments during hemodialysis. The patient suffering from watery diarrhea experiences water loss from the gastrointestinal tract. An increased intake of hypertonic tube feedings may lead to water loss with compartmental fluid shifts. The lungs lose water when a patient suffers from long-term tracheobronchitis or respiratory conditions that cause hyperventilation.

Athletes have the potential to lose several liters of fluid during workout sessions in hot temperatures. When the body's set-point temperature is exceeded to extremes, however, heat cannot be dissipated by sweating or peripheral vasodilation, and heat stroke results.

Problems may also arise when there is an inability to drink water or the situation involves an inactive thirst center. Hypernatremia makes one excessively thirsty; however, patients such as infants or those who are confused or unconscious cannot express this need.

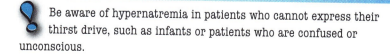

Be aware of hypernatremia in patients who cannot express their thirst drive, such as infants or patients who are confused or unconscious.

Excessive Sodium Intake

Though an excessive intake of dietary sodium is an infrequent cause of hypernatremia, the condition may occur after therapeutic administration of hypertonic intravenous solutions containing sodium. Solutions that include sodium bicarbonate or 3% saline solutions may contribute to increased sodium levels. Corticosteroids may also cause hypernatremia.

MANIFESTATIONS

Mild hypernatremia can essentially go unnoticed. As the situation increases in severity, however, water is lost and the sensation of thirst is triggered. The tongue feels rough and swallowing becomes difficult because the mucous membranes become dry and salivation decreases. The body temperature rises, and the skin becomes warm and flushed. The renal system attempts to conserve fluids, resulting in decreased urine output. However, though the renal system is conserving fluid, the overall fluid volume in the body is low, causing a decrease in blood pressure that causes the heart to work harder and faster.

The most significant effect relates to the central nervous system. When water is pulled from the cells of the central nervous system, dehydration of the brain and nerve cells occurs. The patient initially demonstrates restlessness, irritability, and agitation. Complaints of headache may be present along with seizure activity. Eventually, reflexes decrease and coma results as the hypernatremia progresses (Table 12-2).

Table 12-2 Manifestations of Hypernatremia

Skin	Cardiovascular
Increased temperature, warm, flushed	Decreased blood pressure
Dry mucous membranes	Tachycardia
Difficulty swallowing	Weak, thready pulse
Increased thirst	
Neurological	Renal
Irritability	Decreased urine output
Agitation	
Headache	
Seizures	
Coma	

TREATMENT

Treatment depends on the cause and involves correcting the underlying condition. If the problem is related to a loss of water, treatment begins with replacement of the lost electrolytes and water. The use of glucose–electrolyte solutions given orally are recommended for the less severe conditions. Salt-free solutions, such as 5% dextrose and water, can be administered intravenously if oral intake is compromised. Fluids should be replaced slowly because fluid will now shift to the intracellular compartment, and cerebral edema could result if the shift occurs too rapidly. This is more likely to occur if the hypernatremic condition developed slowly or is chronic. Administering diuretics along with intravenous fluids may also help to decrease sodium levels, but fluid balance must be carefully monitored.

When treating hypernatremia, fluids should be replaced slowly because fluid will now shift to the intracellular compartment, and cerebral edema could result if the shift occurs too rapidly. Fluid balance must be carefully monitored.

Question: What interventions are important for the patient with hypernatremia?

Answer: Monitoring the patient's neurological status, looking for confusion or irritability, vital signs (be alert for low blood pressure, tachycardia, and a weak thready pulse), intake and output, electrolyte status, daily weights, intravenous fluid replacement, and administration of ordered medications. Assess oral membranes and skin integrity.

Conditions resulting in an excessive sodium loss or excessive water gain lead to hyponatremia, a low serum sodium. Hyponatremia results when the serum sodium falls below 135 mEq/L. The serum osmolality also becomes low, falling below 275 mOsm. In this chapter we examine the causes of different types of hyponatremia, hypovolemic and hypervolemic hyponatremia and hypoosmolar and hyperosmolar hyponatremia, and the manifestations these conditions may cause.

13

Hyponatremia

TERMS
- ☐ Hyponatremia
- ☐ Hypervolemic hyponatremia
- ☐ Hypovolemic hyponatremia

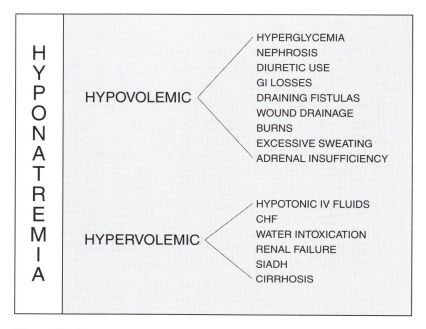

Figure 13-1 Hyponatremia.

CAUSES

Hyponatremia, or low serum sodium, results when the serum sodium falls below 135 mEq/L. The serum osmolality also becomes low, falling below 275 mOsm. In normal renal function the body eliminates excess water by decreasing the release of antidiuretic hormone (see Chapter 8). When this homeostatic mechanism malfunctions, excess water is retained and fluid shifts occur. When more fluid than sodium is present in the intravascular compartment, fluid shifts via osmosis to the more concentrated area inside the cell.

Conditions resulting in an excessive sodium loss or excessive water gain lead to hyponatre-

 Hyponatremia, or low serum sodium, results when the serum sodium falls below 135 mEq/L.

 Conditions resulting in an excessive sodium loss or excessive water gain lead to hyponatremia.

mia. It may also be caused by inadequate sodium intake, although this is atypical and is more likely to occur in patients who are on salt-restricted diets or taking diuretics, such as the elderly.

Hypovolemic Hyponatremia

A dramatic decrease in extracellular fluid volume may lead to excessive sodium loss. This condition, also known as **hypovolemic hyponatremia**, may be caused by nonrenal conditions of excessive loss of gastric secretions from vomiting, diarrhea, gastric suction, or fistulas (Figure 13-1). It may also occur in situations of excessive sweating, wound drainage, or burns. The sodium loss is not necessarily severe unless the fluid loss is replaced with excessive administration of hypotonic intravenous solutions or a large intake of water without electrolyte replacement, both of which produce a dilutional hyponatremia. If the problem is associated with the renal system, the cause may be due to adrenal insufficiency, resulting in a decreased reabsorption of sodium secondary to inadequate levels of aldosterone.

Hypervolemic Hyponatremia

Hypervolemic hyponatremia is the result of an increase in both water and sodium; however, the water gain is more significant. Congestive heart failure, cirrhosis, overuse of hypotonic infusions, and nephritic syndrome can cause hypervolemic hyponatremia (see Figure 13-1).

Hypoosmolar and Hyperosmolar Hyponatremia

Hyponatremia may also be described in relation to osmolality. When the total body water exceeds the normal level of sodium, a hypoosmolar hyponatremia occurs. The syndrome of inappropriate antidiuretic hormone is an example of an abnormal reabsorption of water causing a dilutional hyponatremia with a serum hypoosmolality (see Chapter 43).

Hyperosmolar hyponatremia occurs with increased sugar levels (hyperglycemia). Glucose depends on insulin as a carrier system to cross the cell membrane. In a state of hyperglycemia water shifts from the inside to the outside of the cell, an area of hyperosmolality caused by the increased glucose. Sodium, the major cation outside of the cell, then becomes diluted with the excess water, resulting in hyponatremia despite a condition of hyperosmolality.

MANIFESTATIONS

The manifestations of hyponatremia are related to the fluid shift of water into the cell, resulting in an intracellular swelling and hypoosmolality. The brain and nervous system are the most severely affected. The patient may manifest symptoms of headache, lethargy, and confusion, which may lead to a more serious situation of seizures and coma if serum sodium levels are allowed to fall below 110 mEq/L. If the condition of hyponatremia develops slowly, signs and symptoms of the condition will not be manifested until the serum sodium level reaches approximately 125 mEq/L. Gastrointestinal complaints of abdominal cramps, nausea, vomiting, and diarrhea may also be present.

Patients with hypovolemia demonstrate poor skin turgor, dry cracked mucous membranes, and orthostatic hypotension with a rapid weak pulse. Hemodynamic values may also be decreased. Patients with hypervolemic hyponatremia, however, show evidence of volume overload such as hypertension, a rapid bounding pulse, and elevated hemodynamic values. Pitting edema will be present (Table 13-1).

Table 13-1   Manifestations of Hyponatremia

Neurological	Hypovolemic Hyponatremia
Headache	Poor skin turgor
Lethargy	Dry cracked mucous membranes
Personality change/confusion	Orthostatic hypotension
Absent/diminished reflexes	Rapid weak pulse
Seizures	Decreased hemodynamic values
Coma	
Gastrointestinal	Hypervolemic Hyponatremia
Anorexia	Hypertension
Impaired taste	Rapid bounding pulse
Abdominal cramps	Elevated hemodynamic values
Nausea/vomiting	Pitting edema
Diarrhea	

Question: Why do symptoms of headache, lethargy, and confusion occur with hyponatremia?

Answer: Fluid shifts into the cell, causing intracellular swelling and hypoosmolality. The brain cells are very sensitive to fluid shifts and swell and burst with too much fluid.

TREATMENT

As with any condition, alleviating the underlying cause is the first step toward treatment. If the cause is related to antidiuretic hormone, eliminating medications that may be contributing to the condition will help. Hypervolemic hyponatremia is treated by withholding or restricting fluid intake. Intravenous fluids of normal saline solution may be given to patients with hypovolemic hyponatremia. If the serum sodium is less than 110 mEq/L, a hypertonic solution of 3% or 5% saline may be cautiously administered over a period of time along with loop diuretics to prevent fluid overload.

Whenever a hypertonic solution of saline is administered close attention must be given to the patient to prevent fluid overload. Be alert for signs and symptoms, such as neck vein distension, lung congestion, peripheral edema, or extra heart sounds.

Question: What interventions are important for the patient with hyponatremia?

Answer: Monitor level of consciousness, vital signs, intake and output, lung status, and weight. Oral sodium supplements may be prescribed or fluid restriction.

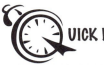

QUICK LOOK AT THE CHAPTER AHEAD

Potassium is the primary intracellular cation regulating intracellular osmolality. Intracellular levels of potassium range from 140 to 150 mEq/L compared with the extracellular level of 3.5 to 5.3 mEq/L. In this chapter we explain the functions of potassium and how it is regulated and maintained.

14

Potassium

TERMS
☐ Potassium

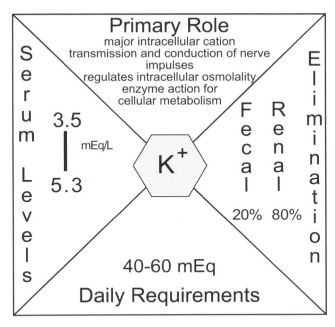

Figure 14-1 Primary role of potassium.

FUNCTIONS

Potassium is the primary intracellular cation, assuming the role of sodium inside the cells and regulating intracellular osmolality. Intracellular levels of potassium range from 140 to 150 mEq/L compared with the extracellular level of 3.5 to 5.3 mEq/L. The

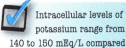

Intracellular levels of potassium range from 140 to 150 mEq/L compared with the extracellular level of 3.5 to 5.3 mEq/L.

sodium–potassium active transport pump is responsible for maintaining this gradient. Primarily regulated by the renal system, 90% of potassium is routinely reabsorbed by the proximal tubule and loop of Henle, with the remainder selectively retained to maintain homeostasis. A normal dietary intake of 40 to 60 mEq allows the average healthy person to balance these losses. Foods such as meats, vegetables, fresh and dried

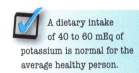

A dietary intake of 40 to 60 mEq of potassium is normal for the average healthy person.

fruits, nuts, and chocolate are good dietary sources. If dietary intake is low, however, or the patient is taking diuretics, potassium may also be supplemented through intravenous fluids or pill or powder supplements. Potassium-sparing diuretics may also help to decrease the total amount of potassium being eliminated from the body. Care should be taken if the patient is receiving multiple transfusions, because potassium is released in stored transfused blood.

 Care should be taken if the patient is receiving multiple whole blood transfusions, because potassium is released in stored transfused blood.

With such a large intracellular stockpile, a small potassium transfer in or out of the cells has a huge effect on blood levels. Safe serum potassium levels have little room for variance. Renal dysfunction, medications, and tissue damage can quickly disrupt this delicate balance. Potassium's effect on maintaining the electrical potential of the cell membrane allows the transmission of nerve impulses and muscle contraction of skeletal and cardiac muscle.

 Safe serum potassium levels have little room for variance. Renal dysfunction, medications, and tissue damage can quickly disrupt this delicate balance.

REGULATION OF POTASSIUM

Potassium is primarily eliminated from the body through renal excretion. Nearly all potassium is filtered at the glomerulus, with selective reabsorption occurring in the proximal tubule and loop of Henle. Variations in glomerular filtration rates as well as hormonal influence determine how much potassium is to be retained. With intact renal function and sufficient free water, the body can adjust filtration rates to maintain homeostasis. When volume is required, sodium is reabsorbed to retain water through osmosis. An inverse relationship exists between sodium and potassium reabsorption in the distal tubules. Dehydration and acute blood loss lead to preferential reabsorption of sodium while leaving potassium in the urine filtrate. When renal function is impaired, excess amounts of potassium build as renal filtration rates decline. Hormonal influences through antidiuretic hormone and aldosterone further modulate reabsorption.

MAINTAINING POTASSIUM BALANCE

Total body stores must be considered but are difficult to estimate from serum levels. Excessive losses may develop slowly through diuretic use or rapidly with profuse diarrhea, depleting body stores. Measurement of these losses is difficult to document and must be anticipated clinically. Potassium shifts out of the cells to replace these losses. Such intracellular changes affect basic cellular functions, such as electric irritability of cardiac muscle. The reverse occurs with overload states, as in renal insufficiency. Reduced excretion can easily drive serum levels beyond tolerance. Release of intracellular potassium from dying cells may be massive, as in the case of crush injuries to muscles or intravascular hemolysis from a transfusion reaction, driving up serum levels.

Shifts between body compartments are often more immediately critical. While diffusion pushes sodium into and potassium out of the cells, active transport pumps are constantly working to maintain the gradient. Any change in the cellular environment influences this delicate balance. Acidosis produces excess hydrogen cations that diffuse throughout all body compartments. As they shift intracellularly, potassium cations must shift out of the cells into the extracellular space to maintain electrical unity. Without altering total body stores, rapid changes in serum potassium levels can occur. Potassium also moves into cells with glucose during active transport. Using intravenous insulin can dangerously lower serum levels in ketoacidosis but can be lifesaving in the initial treatment of severe hyperkalemia.

Questions: If my patient is taking diuretics, what food sources are available to help supplement for lost potassium?

Answer: Dietary sources of potassium are as follows:

- Fruits (oranges, bananas, cantaloupe, apricots)
- Dried fruit
- Vegetables (carrots, mushrooms, tomatoes, potatoes)
- Salt substitutes
- Nuts/seeds
- Chocolate
- Meats

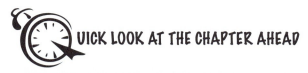

Though the range for a normal potassium level is narrow (3.5–5.3 mEq/L), elevated potassium levels are unusual in the healthy person. Hyperkalemia results when potassium accumulates in the extracellular fluid to a level greater than 5.3 mEq/L. In this chapter we discuss the causes of hyperkalemia, how it is manifested in the body, and treatment.

15

Hyperkalemia

TERMS
☐ **Hyperkalemia**

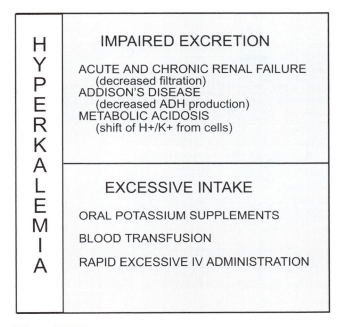

HYPERKALEMIA

IMPAIRED EXCRETION

ACUTE AND CHRONIC RENAL FAILURE
  (decreased filtration)
ADDISON'S DISEASE
  (decreased ADH production)
METABOLIC ACIDOSIS
  (shift of H+/K+ from cells)

EXCESSIVE INTAKE

ORAL POTASSIUM SUPPLEMENTS

BLOOD TRANSFUSION

RAPID EXCESSIVE IV ADMINISTRATION

Figure 15-1 Hyperkalemia: impaired excretion and excessive intake.

CAUSES

Potassium is the main *intracellular* ion. **Hyperkalemia** results when potassium accumulates in the *extracellular* fluid to a level greater than 5.3 mEq/L. Elevated potassium levels are unusual in the healthy person even though the range for a normal potassium level is narrow (3.5–5.3 mEq/L). Potassium becomes elevated in situations of decreased elimination, increased intake, multiple blood transfusions, or with a sudden shift of intracellular potassium to the extracellular compartment (Table 15-1).

The most common cause of hyperkalemia is decreased elimination secondary to renal failure. The renal system is primarily responsible for potassium excretion. When the kidneys are unable to respond to aldosterone (see Chapter 8), the ability to excrete potassium becomes diminished. Certain drugs such as potassium-sparing diuretics, nonsteroidal antiinflammatory drugs, and angiotensin-converting enzyme inhibitors also work by inhibiting aldosterone and contribute to the retention of

Table 15-1 Causes of Hyperkalemia

Renal failure
Multiple blood transfusions
Cellular injury
Acidosis
Diabetic ketoacidosis
Medications
    Potassium-sparing diuretics
    Nonsteroidal antiinflammatory drugs
    Angiotensin-converting enzyme inhibitors
    Digitalis
    Beta-blockers
    Potassium chloride, intravenously or by mouth
    Chemotherapy

potassium. Elevated levels of digitalis inhibit the sodium–potassium pump, thereby inhibiting the balance of electrolytes the pump usually maintains.

Potassium levels can become elevated beyond the normal range with rapid intravenous administration of potassium chloride, particularly in the patient with compromised renal function. Lethal results occur when intravenous potassium is given directly without dilution. Potassium should never be given in this manner but should always be diluted with the recommended amount of an intravenous solution.

Lethal results occur when intravenous potassium is given directly without dilution. Potassium should never be given in this manner but should always be diluted with the recommended amount of an intravenous solution and administered via an infusion pump.

Cells that are crushed from injury or burns release intracellular potassium to the extracellular compartment. Potassium also moves from the intracellular fluid compartment to the extracellular fluid compartment during a state of acidosis as the hydrogen ion is exchanged for the potassium ion or with a change in cell membrane permeability with situations causing hypoxia. Insulin

Potassium moves from the intracellular fluid compartment to the extracellular fluid compartment during a state of acidosis as the hydrogen ion is exchanged for the potassium ion.

is responsible for facilitating transportation of potassium into the cell; therefore insulin deficits such as those occurring in diabetes mellitus may also result in hyperkalemia.

MANIFESTATIONS

The manifestations associated with an elevated potassium level sometimes involve the smooth muscles, which becomes hypopolarized. This affects the gastrointestinal system, initiating early symptoms of nausea, cramping, and diarrhea (Table 15-2). A more common manifestation, however, is the effect on neuromuscular function. As the potassium level rises, the muscle cells become increasingly hypopolarized so that the resting membrane potential lies above the threshold potential. This results in an inability of the cell to contract once it has discharged and the outcome can result in paresthesias, muscle weakness, and flaccid paralysis. The effect tends to start in the lower extremities and spreads to the trunk and eventually to the respiratory muscles.

The most serious effect of hyperkalemia, however, results in cardiac arrest. Dangerous dysrhythmias begin to develop when the serum potassium level reaches 7.0 mEq/L. Like the skeletal muscle, the cardiac muscle cells also become hypopolarized. The action potential and conduction velocity are decreased, resulting in dysrhythmias, some potentially lethal. The electrocardiogram shows changes with the P wave, representative of atrial depolarization, becoming flattened. The PR interval becomes prolonged, indicating a delay between conduction of the atria to the ventricles. The QRS complex widens, representing a depressed depolarization of the ventricular muscle cell; the T segment becomes tall and peaked;

Table 15-2 Manifestations of Hyperkalemia

Neurological	Gastrointestinal
Vague muscle weakness	Abdominal cramping
Paresthesias	Nausea
Flaccid paralysis	Diarrhea
Respiratory	Cardiovascular
Respiratory depression	Bradycardia
from muscle weakness	Heart block
	Ventricular fibrillation
	Cardiac arrest

and the ST segment becomes depressed, indicating a prolonged depolarization of the ventricular cardiac muscle (Figure 15-2).

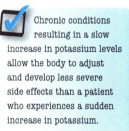

Chronic conditions resulting in a slow increase in potassium levels allow the body to adjust and develop less severe side effects than a patient who experiences a sudden increase in potassium.

The clinical manifestations may vary in individuals depending on the cause and rapidity of the elevation of potassium. Chronic conditions resulting in a slow increase in potassium levels allow the body to adjust and develop less severe side effects than a patient who experiences a sudden increase in potassium. Patients undergoing a rapid rise are more likely to manifest the neuromuscular symptoms.

HYPERKALEMIC EFFECT ON ECG

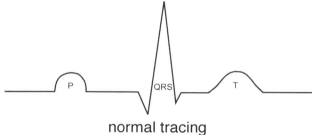

normal tracing
(K^+ levels between 3.5-5.3 mEq/L)

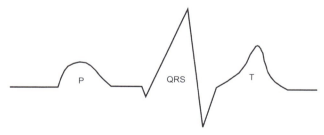

tall peaked T Wave, prolonged PR interval, depressed ST segment, QRS wider with $K^+ > 7$ mEq/L

Figure 15-2   Hyperkalemic effect on the electrocardiogram.

TREATMENT

Treatment depends on the cause and severity of the hyperkalemia. Patients with chronic renal failure should be taught about the hidden dietary sources of potassium. In particular, certain salt substitutes contain large amounts of potassium and should be restricted in this client. Dialysis will help to eliminate high potassium levels in acute and chronic conditions. In emergency situations a combination of insulin and glucose may temporarily help to move potassium into the cell. Kayexalate, a sodium polystyrene sulfonate combined with sorbitol, may be given orally or rectally as a retention enema. Potassium is removed via the loose stool as it is replaced with sodium, which moves into the blood in exchange for potassium's movement into the intestine.

Patients with chronic renal failure should be taught about the hidden dietary sources of potassium. In particular, certain salt substitutes contain large amounts of potassium and should be restricted in this client.

Question: What interventions are important for the patient with hyperkalemia?

Answer: Be alert for muscle weakness with the extremities or hypermotility in the gastrointestinal tract. Assess for an irregular pulse, decreased heart rate, and low blood pressure.

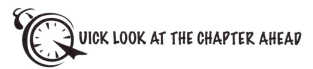

A serum level of potassium below 3.5 mEq/L is considered hypokalemia. A low potassium level results from an inadequate intake, excessive loss, or a shift of potassium from the extracellular compartment to the intracellular compartment. The loss of potassium through such events generally takes place slowly over time. Here we discuss the causes, manifestations, and treatment of hypokalemia.

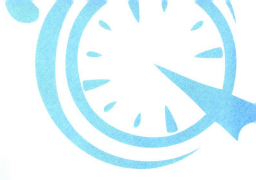

16

Hypokalemia

TERMS
☐ **Hypokalemia**

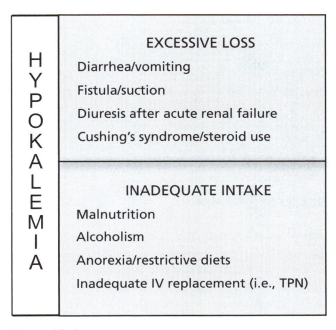

H Y P O K A L E M I A	**EXCESSIVE LOSS** Diarrhea/vomiting Fistula/suction Diuresis after acute renal failure Cushing's syndrome/steroid use
	INADEQUATE INTAKE Malnutrition Alcoholism Anorexia/restrictive diets Inadequate IV replacement (i.e., TPN)

Figure 16-1 Hypokalemia: excessive loss and inadequate intake.

CAUSES

Hypokalemia is defined as a serum level of potassium below 3.5 mEq/L. When an inadequate intake, excessive loss, or a shift of potassium from the extracellular compartment to the intracellular compartment occurs, a low potassium level results.

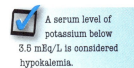
A serum level of potassium below 3.5 mEq/L is considered hypokalemia.

Decreased Intake of Potassium

Insufficient potassium intake can occur from an improper diet. Fad diets or administration of large amounts of potassium-deficient intravenous fluids could result in hypokalemia (Table 16-1).

Table 16-1 Causes of Hypokalemia

Improper diet (i.e., fad diets, potassium-deficient intravenous fluids)
Medications (i.e., diuretics, laxatives)
Congestive heart failure
Gastrointestinal (i.e., suction, vomiting, diarrhea, fistulas)
Liver diseases
Hyperaldosteronism
Nephritis
Steroids
Cushing's syndrome

Excessive Loss of Potassium

A large loss of potassium could occur with excessive use of diuretics. Potassium is lost via urine. Overuse of diuretics or use of diuretics that are too potent without potassium supplementation could result in hypokalemia. Intestinal fluids are also rich in potassium. Laxative abuse or loss of fluids through the gastrointestinal system due to suction, vomiting, diarrhea, or fistulas can lead to a loss of potassium. Insulin, which shifts potassium into the cell; corticosteroids; and certain antibiotics can also be responsible for depleting potassium from the body.

Compartment Shifts

Conditions such as excessive gastric suctioning or vomiting can lead to alkalosis. During alkalosis the hydrogen ion exits the cell in exchange for the potassium ion that enters the cell, causing an artificial loss of potassium. Other conditions such as hyperaldosteronism, congestive heart failure, diseases of the liver, and nephritis may lead to a hypokalemic state.

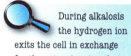

During alkalosis the hydrogen ion exits the cell in exchange for the potassium ion that enters the cell, causing an artificial loss of potassium.

MANIFESTATIONS

Hypokalemia is known for causing an altered function of skeletal and smooth muscle, allowing the muscle to become hyperpolarized and less reactive to stimuli. A mild case of hypokalemia may start as bilateral muscle weakness, starting in the lower extremities with leg cramps and paresthesias. If the potassium loss progresses, flaccid paralysis may occur. The complications ascend up the body, affecting the smooth muscle. The gastrointestinal system may be affected, with diminished bowel function resulting in abdominal distention and possible paralytic ileus (Table 16-2). An extreme complication of respiratory paralysis may occur, but this happens infrequently.

The cardiac muscle cells initially become hyperpolarized with decreased potassium levels, but as the levels become dangerously low the cells become hypopolarized, resulting in an increased diastolic depolarization. This results in excitability of the cells and the development of ectopic beats. Decreased conduction velocity of impulses through the atrioventricular node and prolonging of the cardiac action potential occur. Such effects on the heart present as a weak and irregular pulse along with orthostatic hypotension. The electrocardiogram may show a depressed ST segment, flattened T wave, and a U wave (Figure 16-2). The ectopic beats that irritate the ventricle may potentiate lethal dysrhythmias and eventual cardiac arrest. Hypokalemia especially affects the patient on digitalis glycosides, increasing the risk for digitalis toxicity.

Question: **What happens to the cardiac muscle when the patient is hypokalemic?**

Answer: **Hypokalemia's effects on the heart may cause a weak and irregular pulse along with orthostatic hypotension. The ectopic beats that irritate the ventricle may potentiate lethal dysrhythmias and eventual cardiac arrest.**

Table 16-2 Manifestations of Hypokalemia

Neuromuscular	Gastrointestinal
Bilateral extremity muscle weakness	Diminished bowel function
Paresthesias	Abdominal distention
Hyporeflexia	Paralytic ileus
Leg cramps	Constipation
Cardiovascular	Renal
Weak irregular pulse	Polyuria
Hypotension	
Electrocardiogram changes	
Lethal dysrhythmias	
Cardiac arrest	

HYPOKALEMIC EFFECT ON ECG

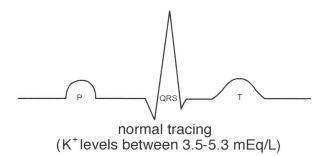

normal tracing
(K^+ levels between 3.5-5.3 mEq/L)

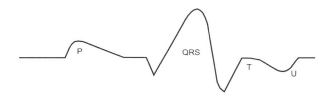

depressed ST segment, T wave
inversion, U waves (K^+ level <3.5 mEq/L)

Figure 16-2   Hypokalemic effect on the electrocardiogram.

 Hypokalemia especially affects the patient on digitalis glycosides, increasing the risk for digitalis toxicity.

Question: What interventions are important for the patient with hypokalemia?

Answer: Follow acid–base balance, assessing for signs of irritability and paresthesias related to a state of alkalosis. Assess cardiac status, monitoring heart rate and rhythm for irregularities. Assess respiratory rate for weakness or distress. Document intake and output and monitor electrolyte status closely. Follow strict guidelines for replacing potassium via intravenous lines.

TREATMENT

Treatment involves replacing the lost potassium. Monitoring serum laboratory values determines the severity of the condition. If the situation is a mild loss of potassium, oral supplements may help raise the level. If the loss is more severe, intravenous potassium administration may be necessary. Intravenous potassium is always diluted with intravenous solutions according to guidelines for recommended concentrations. It is never given undiluted in an intravenous push or bolus, because administering potassium in this manner results in cardiac arrest.

Intravenous potassium is always diluted with intravenous solutions according to guidelines for recommended concentrations, mixed well, and administered via an intravenous infusion pump. It is never given undiluted in an intravenous push or bolus, because administering potassium in this manner results in cardiac arrest.

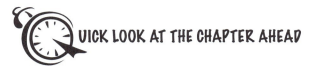

Calcium is a mineral that helps to build and maintain the bones and teeth, regulate the heart's rhythm, transmit nerve impulses, and assist with blood clotting. The body gets calcium through food sources and by borrowing it from the bones when calcium blood levels are low. The normal range for total serum calcium is 8.5–10.5 mg/dL or 4.5–5.5 mEq/L. In this chapter we describe the functions of calcium and how it is regulated and maintained.

17

Calcium

TERMS
☐ **Calcium**

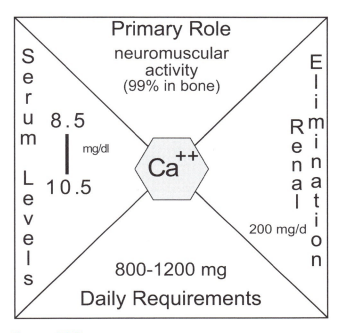

Figure 17-1 Primary role of calcium.

FUNCTION

The normal range for total serum calcium is 8.5–10.5 mg/dL or 4.5–5.5 mEq/L. Ninety-nine percent of calcium is located in the bones and teeth and is responsible for the formation and firm structure of these body parts. This leaves 1% of calcium in the cells and fluid compartments, with the majority of that 1% in the extracellular compartment. Forty-one percent of this extracellular calcium is bound to the protein albumin. Therefore when albumin levels decline, so do calcium levels. A small percentage is bound to citrate and other small organic ions. The remainder of calcium is ionized (unbound). The

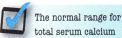 The normal range for total serum calcium is 8.5–10.5 mg/dL or 4.5–5.5 mEq/L.

 Ninety-nine percent of calcium is located in the bones and teeth, leaving 1% of calcium in the cells and fluid compartments.

normal value for ionized calcium is 4.5–5.1 mg/dL or 2.2–2.5 mEq/L. This ionized or free calcium conducts the physiological functions, and any imbalances in the levels of ionized calcium result in hypocalcemia or hypercalcemia. Calcium functions in cellular permeability and in the contraction of cardiac, smooth, and skeletal muscles. It also plays a role in the blood-clotting process.

REGULATION OF CALCIUM

Calcium is ingested through food sources, especially dairy products and green leafy vegetables (Table 17-1). It is absorbed from the small intestine, and elimination occurs in the urine and feces. The minimum daily requirement is 800–1,200 mg/day. This amount varies, however, with pregnancy, childhood, and conditions of osteoporosis. When calcium levels are low, parathyroid hormone helps to regulate calcium by mobilizing it, pulling it out of the bones, and releasing it into the bloodstream. In an effort to replace borrowed calcium, this hormone also dictates kidney reabsorption and along with vitamin D promotes intestinal absorption of calcium in an effort to maintain regulation. In contrast to parathyroid hormone, calcitonin, secreted by the thyroid gland,

 When serum calcium levels are low, the body has a banking system of borrowing calcium from the bones in an effort to increase serum calcium levels. Calcium is borrowed with the intention that the body will repay or restore these levels at a later date. However, after the age of 30 bone destruction tends to exceed bone rebuilding, and caution must be taken to attempt to keep levels from getting too low. Therefore, in addition to consuming enough calcium, regularly performing weight-bearing exercises and taking care to obtain adequate amounts of vitamins D and K are of vital importance.

Table 17-1 Calcium Food Sources

Milk, yogurt, cheese, ice cream, tofu
Canned salmon, sardines
Broccoli, turnip greens, Chinese cabbage, kale
Rhubarb
Pinto beans
Almonds
Figs
Calcium-fortified fruit juices and drinks, some cereals

regulates elevated calcium levels by increasing calcium deposits in the bone, decreasing gastrointestinal absorption, and increasing renal elimination of calcium.

MAINTAINING CALCIUM BALANCE

The extracellular levels of calcium are kept in balance in the healthy individual through dietary intake and reabsorption from bone and kidney. Vitamin D is essential for absorption of calcium from the available sources. An increased intake of calcium will not raise blood levels or be properly absorbed without vitamin D, which is easily obtained through sunshine and food sources such as dairy products. Vitamin K, also important for calcium regulation and the formation of bone, can be found primarily in green leafy vegetables.

Question: **What type of food sources supply calcium?**

Answer: **Dairy products, such as milk, yogurt, and cheese, are the biggest sources of calcium intake. For those who are lactose intolerant or choose not to eat animals or animal products, other calcium food sources exist (see Table 17-1).**

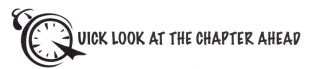

Hypercalcemia is documented when the serum calcium level rises above 10.5 mg/dL or 5.5 mEq/L. It has few specific findings to its diagnosis. Symptoms tend to overlap those of an underlying disease or cancerous condition. In this chapter we take a closer look at the causes, manifestations, and treatment of hypercalcemia.

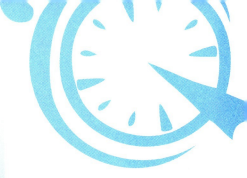

18

Hypercalcemia

TERMS
- [ ] **Hypercalcemia**

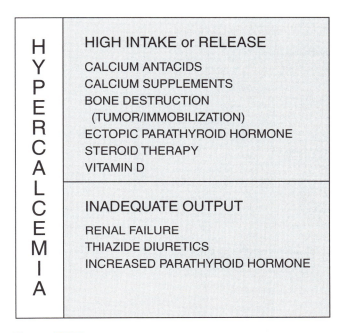

| H
Y
P
E
R
C
A
L
C
E
M
I
A | **HIGH INTAKE or RELEASE**

CALCIUM ANTACIDS
CALCIUM SUPPLEMENTS
BONE DESTRUCTION
  (TUMOR/IMMOBILIZATION)
ECTOPIC PARATHYROID HORMONE
STEROID THERAPY
VITAMIN D |
| | **INADEQUATE OUTPUT**

RENAL FAILURE
THIAZIDE DIURETICS
INCREASED PARATHYROID HORMONE |

Figure 18-1 High intake or release and inadequate output.

CAUSES

Hypercalcemia results when the movement of calcium into the circulation overwhelms the ability of the regulatory hormones or the renal system to eliminate excess calcium ions. Hypercalcemia is documented when the serum calcium level rises above 10.5 mg/dL or 5.5 mEq/L. Ionized serum calcium levels must rise above 5.25 mg/dL or 2.5 mEq/L for hypercalcemia to exist.

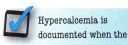 Hypercalcemia is documented when the serum calcium level rises above 10.5 mg/dL or 5.5 mEq/L. Ionized serum calcium levels must rise above 5.25 mg/dL or 2.5 mEq/L for hypercalcemia to exist.

Hyperparathyroidism can be responsible for hypercalcemia due to the increased production of parathyroid hormone, which helps activate calcium from bone (Table 18-1). Another cause for hypercalcemia is the destruction of bone secondary to malignant cells of certain cancers, such

Table 18-1   Causes of Hypercalcemia

Hyperparathyroidism
Hypophosphatemia
Cancers
    Lung
    Breast
    Ovary
    Prostate
    Gastrointestinal
    Leukemia
Prolonged immobilization
Multiple fractures
Medications
    Thiazide diuretics
    Steroids
    Calcium supplements and antacids
Vitamin D

as lung, breast, ovary, prostate, gastrointestinal, and leukemia. Often, the symptoms of hypercalcemia mimic those of the malignancy. The patient seeks medical attention for the symptoms of the undiagnosed malignancy and at the same time receives the diagnosis of hypercalcemia.

Less common causes of hypercalcemia are prolonged immobility or multiple fractures leading to demineralization and the release of calcium from bone. Excessive vitamin D or calcium-containing supplements can lead to an increased intestinal absorption of calcium. A decreased excretion of calcium by the kidneys through the use of thiazide diuretics can result in hypercalcemia. Thiazide diuretics are also known for promoting the action of parathyroid hormone, helping to increase calcium reabsorption. Phosphorus is known to inhibit calcium absorption in the intestines; therefore hypophosphatemia is related to hypercalcemia. The serum pH also has an inverse relationship with ionized calcium. As the pH level drops, resulting in acidosis, less calcium binds to protein, causing an increased ionized calcium level.

 Calcium levels do not have to be seriously elevated to affect the elderly patient; the elderly patient is more likely to be symptomatic from calcium levels that are moderately elevated.

MANIFESTATIONS

Calcium functions in the contraction of cardiac, skeletal, and smooth muscles, and hypercalcemia causes a decrease in cell membrane excitability. The heart muscle may respond through increased contractility demonstrated on the electrocardiogram as a shortened QT interval decreased or diminished ST segment. Ventricular dysrhythmias, bradyarrhythmias, and heart block may develop into asystole (Table 18-2). If the patient is taking digitalis, the responses to these conditions may be accentuated.

Neural excitability decreases with hypercalcemia, allowing for a change in personality or a dulling of consciousness, stupor, and possible coma in more severe cases. Patients may complain of fatigue and muscle weakness. Muscle tone becomes decreased and a hyporeflexia develops.

As a result of the smooth muscle being affected, gastrointestinal symptoms of anorexia, nausea, vomiting, and constipation develop. Stones may develop, causing a blocking of the pancreatic ducts, resulting in pancreatitis.

The renal system is responsible for concentrating urine; however, in situations involving hypercalcemia, the high levels of calcium interfere with the action of antidiuretic hormone, causing diuresis and subsequent dehydration. Renal calculi can also occur due to elevated calcium levels.

Hypercalcemic crisis is the result of an acute situation generally stemming from malignant disease or hyperparathyroidism. This condition

Table 18-2 Manifestations of Hypercalcemia

Cardiac	Gastrointestinal
Ventricular dysrhythmias	Anorexia
Bradyarrhythmias	Nausea/vomiting
Heart block	Constipation
Asystole	Abdominal or flank pain
	Pancreatitis
Neural	Renal
Personality changes, psychosis, confusion	Calculi
Decreased memory	Polyuria
Headache	Dehydration
Stupor, possible coma	
Lethargy, muscle weakness	
Depressed reflexes	

results in polyuria, which contributes to a state of dehydration; excessive thirst; fever; azotemia (a collection of nitrogenous waste products); altered level of consciousness; and cardiac arrest. This rapid chain of events usually results in a high mortality rate.

TREATMENT

Hypercalcemia is treated by correcting the underlying problem, keeping calcium from leaving bone, and allowing for renal excretion. Patients with chronic kidney disease should undergo dialysis. For others, sodium and calcium are eliminated together; therefore the combination of a normal saline solution and calcitonin can be rapidly administered followed by a loop diuretic such as Lasix. This combination helps with a rapid dilution and diuresis of calcium. Rehydration is also important and must be closely monitored when diuresis is part of the treatment.

Loop diuretics are recommended for treatment of hypercalcemia as opposed to thiazide diuretics, which increase the reabsorption of calcium.

Bisphosphonates and calcitonin are drugs that inhibit bone reabsorption through inhibition of osteoclastic activity. Plicamycin (mithramycin) and corticosteroids help to inhibit bone reabsorption for cancer patients. Plicamycin is nephrotoxic and hepatotoxic and therefore should be used with caution in long-term patients.

Question: What interventions are important for the patient with hypercalcemia?

Answer: Monitor vital signs and assess for cardiac dysrhythmias that may develop. Monitor intake and output, administering diuretics and fluid as needed. Monitor electrolyte levels closely. Encourage ambulation for prevention of calcium release from the bone and to assist peristalsis in the event of renal calculi.

QUICK LOOK AT THE CHAPTER AHEAD

Normal calcium exchange in the blood is controlled by the parathyroid hormone. Hypocalcemia results when the calcium level falls below 8.5 mg/dL or 4.5 mEq/L. Hypocalcemic states occur through excessive loss of calcium from the body, either from a lack of ingestion or absorption of the mineral. In this chapter we discuss the many causes of hypocalcemia as well as manifestations and treatment.

19

Hypocalcemia

TERMS
- [ ] **Chvostek's sign**
- [ ] **Hypoalbuminemia**
- [ ] **Hypocalcemia**
- [ ] **Trousseau's sign**

```
H   INADEQUATE INTAKE
Y   VITAMIN DEFICIENCY
P
O   POOR DIETARY CALCIUM SOURCES
C
A   ALCOHOLISM
L
C   LIMITS ABSORPTION
E   (MEDICATIONS / CHRONIC DIARRHEA)
M
I   EXCESSIVE LOSSES
A   PRIMARY/SECONDARY
    HYPOPARATHYROIDISM
    RENAL FAILURE AND/OR
    HIGH PHOSPHATE
    ALKALOSIS
    (INCREASES PROTEIN BINDING)
    PANCREATITIS
    LAXATIVES
```

Figure 19-1 Inadequate intake and excessive losses.

CAUSES

Normally, calcium is extracted from the bone and replaced on a daily basis. In addition, the amount of calcium that is absorbed from the intestine is matched by that excreted through the kidneys. All of this calcium exchange is controlled by the parathyroid hormone. **Hypocalcemia** results when the calcium level falls below 8.5 mg/dL or 4.5 mEq/L. Hypocalcemic states occur through excessive loss of calcium from the body, from either a lack of ingestion or absorption of the mineral. Alcoholics are particularly prone to developing hypocalcemia secondary to a lack of intake and poor absorption related to a malnourished state (Table 19-1).

Pancreatitis can result in hypocalcemia due to a decreased absorption and an increased excretion of calcium. Pancreatitis results in a decrease in pancreatic lipase, which normally helps with the digestion of

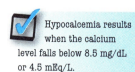

Hypocalcemia results when the calcium level falls below 8.5 mg/dL or 4.5 mEq/L.

Table 19-1 Causes of Hypocalcemia

Alcoholism	Hypoalbuminemia secondary to
Pancreatitis	Cirrhosis
Gastrointestinal problems	Malnutrition
Prolonged diarrhea	Nephrosis
Overuse of laxatives	Burns
Chronic renal failure	Chronic illness
Decreased parathyroid hormone	Sepsis
Hyperphosphatemia	
Medications	
Mithramycin	
Calcitonin	
Diuretics	
Cisplatin	
Gentamicin	

dietary fats. Because the fats cannot be absorbed, calcium from the diet and that secreted into the intestine cannot be absorbed. Instead, calcium is bound to the undigested fat and excreted from the body.

Malabsorption of calcium occurs when the ion cannot be absorbed properly in the gastrointestinal tract. Situations of prolonged diarrhea, overuse of laxatives, or increased intestinal motility result in malabsorption. Calcium needs vitamin D for proper absorption, and when certain medications, such as anticonvulsants, interfere with vitamin D metabolism, calcium absorption suffers. Chronic renal failure also can be the cause of poor absorption of calcium as the kidneys lose the ability to activate vitamin D.

Parathyroid hormone, which is responsible for kidney reabsorption and intestinal absorption of calcium, can be the cause of hypocalcemia if the parathyroid gland is removed. Thyroid surgery, hypomagnesemia, hypoparathyroidism, and tumors of or injury to the parathyroid gland can all result in reduced or a complete lack of parathyroid hormone. Another cause of hypocalcemia is high phosphorus levels (hyperphosphatemia) found in critically ill patients. Phosphate binds with calcium, causing hypocalcemia.

Mithramycin and calcitonin are drugs known for decreased calcium resorption from bone. Diuretics, particularly the loop diuretics such as furosemide (Lasix) or ethacrynic acid (Edecrin), can bring about hypocalcemia by eliminating the ion through an increased urine output.

Phosphates or drugs that lower serum magnesium, such as cisplatin or gentamicin, can also contribute to a low calcium level.

Because 41% of calcium binds to protein, when protein (albumin) stores are low (hypoalbuminemia) calcium levels also drop. **Hypoalbuminemia** is the most common cause of hypocalcemia and results from numerous causes, including cirrhosis, malnutrition, nephrosis, burns, many different types of chronic illnesses, or sepsis.

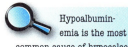

Hypoalbuminemia is the most common cause of hypocalcemia. Because 41% of calcium binds to protein, when protein (albumin) stores are low (hypoalbuminemia) calcium levels also drop.

MANIFESTATIONS

Calcium is important for determining the speed of ion fluxes, causing muscle contraction; therefore as hypercalcemia causes decreased muscle contraction and excitability, hypocalcemia causes increased muscle contraction and excitability. Action potentials of the muscle cell are easily generated with hypocalcemia. This excitability increases to the point of neuromuscular irritability manifested by a positive Chvostek's or Trousseau's sign, muscle twitching, paresthesias, and cramping, leading to potential tetany (Table 19-2). Hyperactive reflexes may develop along with seizures. Cardiac dysrhythmias result from a prolonged plateau phase of the cardiac action potential (prolonged QT). This affects atrioventricular and intraventricular conduction as well as myocardial contractility.

Table 19-2　Manifestations of Hypocalcemia

Anxiety, confusion, depression, irritability
Fatigue/lethargy
Numbness/tingling around mouth and extremities/toes/fingers
Hyperreflexia
Twitching, jitteriness, tremors, muscle cramps
Chvostek's sign
Trousseau's sign
Tetany
Laryngeal spasm
Seizures
Cardiac dysrhythmias

Trousseau's and Chvostek's Signs

Testing for a positive **Trousseau's sign** can be done by occluding arterial blood flow with an inflated blood pressure cuff above systolic pressure on the upper arm for approximately 3 minutes. If this is followed by a carpal spasm (flexed wrist and metacarpophalangeal joints, extended interphalangeal joints, and adducted thumb) the test is

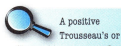

A positive Trousseau's or Chvostek's sign are reflective of increased neuromuscular irritability and may be indicative of hypocalcemia but should be interpreted with caution.

positive for increased neuromuscular irritability. Tapping the facial nerve in front of the ear may produce a spasm or brief contraction of the corner of the mouth, nose, eye, and muscles in the cheek, which is considered to be a positive **Chvostek's sign**. This is a graded response depending on the calcium level. Though these tests are reflective of increased neuromuscular irritability that may relate to hypocalcemia, they also may point to other conditions and should be interpreted with caution.

TREATMENT

Treatment depends on the underlying cause and treating the primary source of the problem. If the situation is acute, intravenous calcium gluconate or calcium chloride may be given. Vitamin D may be given to help absorption of oral calcium supplements in the gastrointestinal tract if the condition becomes chronic.

Question: What interventions are important for the patient with hypocalcemia?

Answer: Assess vital signs and evaluate for a positive Trousseau's or Chvostek's sign. Assess respiratory status and be alert for dyspnea or stridor. Maintain a tracheotomy tray and Ambu-bag at bedside in case of laryngospasm and the need for an emergency tracheotomy. Monitor cardiac status for dysrhythmias. Administer intravenous calcium supplements with extreme caution, preferably through a central line. Administer oral supplements approximately 1 hour after eating.

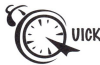

Chloride is a mineral electrolyte, found primarily in the extracellular fluid, that helps distribute body fluids by attaching to sodium or water. In the stomach it joins with the hydrogen ion to form hydrochloric acid. Serum chloride levels range between 98 and 106 mEq/L in the extracellular fluid and approximately 4 mEq/L in the intracellular fluid. In this chapter we discuss the function of chloride, its regulation, and how its balance is maintained in the body.

20

Chloride

TERMS
☐ **Chloride**

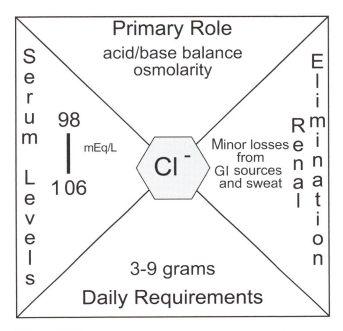

Figure 20-1 Primary role and daily requirements of chloride.

FUNCTION

Serum **chloride** levels range between 98 and 106 mEq/L in the extracellular fluid and approximately 4 mEq/L in the intracellular fluid. Chloride, the most abundant anion in the extracellular fluid, can be found in gastric secretions, pancreatic juices, and bile. It is most plentiful in the cerebrospinal fluid, where it joins with sodium. Its negative charge allows it to bind and travel with the positively charged ions of sodium, potassium, calcium, and others.

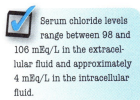

Serum chloride levels range between 98 and 106 mEq/L in the extracellular fluid and approximately 4 mEq/L in the intracellular fluid.

Bound with sodium, the combination forms sodium chloride, responsible for maintaining fluid balance and osmolality. When sodium and chloride are retained, so is water; when sodium and chloride are lost through the renal system, water also is lost. When the osmolality is increased, more sodium and chloride ions are available compared with the percentage of water. When the osmolality is decreased, the number of sodium and chloride ions is also decreased compared with the percentage of water.

In the digestive system chloride forms with the hydrogen ion to make hydrochloric acid, aiding in digestion. It also plays an important role in maintaining acid–base balance.

REGULATION OF CHLORIDE

Most of the required daily intake of chloride (3–9 g) is obtained through a healthy diet. This most commonly occurs through the use of table salt. However, chloride is also found in fruits, vegetables, cheese, milk, eggs, fish, and as a hidden source in canned vegetables or processed meats (Table 20-1). It is easily absorbed by the small intestine and eliminated via the kidneys or through the skin with heavy perspiration.

Patients on low-sodium diets should be taught about the hidden sources of chloride in canned or processed foods as well as in salt substitutes (KCl).

MAINTAINING CHLORIDE BALANCE

Chloride is transported passively and, due to its affinity for sodium, follows the active transport of sodium. Therefore chloride levels in the body are increased or decreased proportionally along with changes in the

Table 20-1 Dietary Sources of Chloride

Table salt and sea salt
Vegetables (i.e., spinach, celery, lettuce, tomatoes)
Fish
Fruits (i.e., dates, bananas)
Dairy products (i.e., cheese, milk, eggs)
Processed meats and foods
Soy sauce
Seaweed (i.e., kelp)
Olives
Rye

sodium level. Sodium is directly affected by aldosterone, which indirectly affects chloride's relationship with sodium. As aldosterone is secreted, sodium is reabsorbed by the kidneys and chloride becomes passively reabsorbed as it attaches itself to the sodium ion.

Chloride is exchanged for HCO_3 as the body maintains its acid–base balance. HCO_3 is retained to increase alkalinity, and chloride is excreted. When the body needs a more acidic balance, HCO_3 is excreted via the kidneys and chloride is retained (see Chapter 30).

Question: Should we look for additional foods to supplement chloride in our diet?

Answer: No, our diets are already high in salt content, and most people consume enough salt to satisfy the body's requirement for chloride.

Hyperchloremia is an excess amount of chloride in the blood. A level exceeding 106 mEq/L in the extracellular fluid constitutes a hyperchloremic condition. A hyperchloremic imbalance is usually due to an underlying condition, without signs and symptoms of its own. Here we define the causes, manifestations, and treatment for this electrolyte disorder.

21

Hyperchloremia

TERMS
- [ ] **Hyperchloremia**

<table>
<tr><td rowspan="2">H Y P E R C H L O R E M I A</td><td>**INCREASED INTAKE/EXCHANGE**

EXCESS SALT INTAKE WITHOUT WATER

HYPERTONIC IV FLUID ADMINISTRATION

METABOLIC ACIDOSIS</td></tr>
<tr><td>**DECREASED LOSSES**

HYPERPARATHYROIDISM

HYPERALDOSTERONISM

RENAL FAILURE</td></tr>
</table>

Figure 21-1 Increased intake exchange and decreased losses.

CAUSES

Hyperchloremia is an excess amount of chloride in the blood. A level exceeding 106 mEq/L in the extracellular fluid constitutes a hyperchloremic condition. Chloride has an affinity for sodium and an inverse relationship with bicarbonate. These relationships

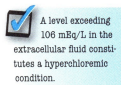

A level exceeding 106 mEq/L in the extracellular fluid constitutes a hyperchloremic condition.

are reflected in a chloride imbalance. High levels of chloride are related to excess sodium or decreased bicarbonate levels in the body. In addition, the renal system controls the elimination of chloride from the body; therefore an imbalance with serum chloride levels may be related to kidney disfunction.

Hyperchloremia can result from an increased intake orally or via administration of hypertonic intravenous fluids of sodium chloride coupled with a loss of water. Because of chloride's inverse relationship with bicarbonate, hyperchloremia occurs in conditions of metabolic acidosis, when serum bicarbonate levels are low (see Chapter 30). Endocrine conditions such as hyperparathyroidism, hyperaldosteronism, or diabetes insipidus may be the cause of hyperchloremia, as well as hypernatremia, due to the ability of chloride to bind with sodium (Table 21-1).

Certain drugs that contain chloride can be responsible for elevated chloride blood levels. Salicylate toxicity may cause hyperchloremia. Kayexalate, an ion exchange resin, is used in conditions of hyperkalemia and works by exchanging potassium for chloride in the bowel, eliminating the potassium and retaining chloride.

MANIFESTATIONS

Hyperchloremia does not cause signs and symptoms related to a high chloride level. This electrolyte imbalance is usually due to an underlying condition; therefore the manifestations are related to that particular condition (Table 21-2). The chloride level is usually elevated when the sodium is high (i.e., hypernatremia), and the signs and symptoms would then relate to fluid overload (see Table 9-1). The heart rate may be tachycardic, blood pressure may be elevated, and dyspnea may be experienced, all secondary to excess fluid.

Be alert for an elevated chloride level along with signs of fluid overload (i.e., agitation, edema, distended neck veins, tachypnea, dyspnea, hypertension, and tachycardia).

Table 21-1   Causes of Hyperchloremia

Metabolic acidosis
Hyperparathyroidism
Hyperaldosteronism
Hypernatremia
Renal disorders, renal failure
Diabetes insipidus
Dehydration
Medications (i.e., salicylate toxicity, ion exchange resins)

Table 21-2 Manifestations of Hyperchloremia

Inverse relationship of chloride and HCO_3 = hyperchloremic acidosis secondary to HCO_3 loss
Metabolic acidosis
    Lethargy
    Weakness
    Decreased level of consciousness
    Tachypnea
    Kussmaul's respiration
Hyperchloremia secondary to hypernatremia
    Edema
    Distended neck veins
    Agitation
    Tachypnea
    Dyspnea
    Hypertension
    Tachycardia

Similarly, if hyperchloremia is due to an acidotic state, the signs and symptoms would be related to the acidotic state, not to the hyperchloremia. Signs and symptoms related to acidosis would be tachypnea, along with neurological manifestations of weakness, lethargy, and decreased cognition.

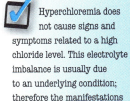 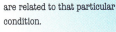 Hyperchloremia does not cause signs and symptoms related to a high chloride level. This electrolyte imbalance is usually due to an underlying condition; therefore the manifestations are related to that particular condition.

TREATMENT

Treatment involves correcting the underlying condition. If hypernatremia is the cause, administering diuretics to assist in eliminating sodium also helps in removal of the chloride ion.

In states of acidosis administering bicarbonate helps to correct the acidotic state, and through competition for the connection with sodium, chloride is eliminated. Lactated Ringer's solution may also be administered to help increase the bicarbonate level because the liver converts the lactate to bicarbonate.

Question: What interventions are important for the patient with hyperchloremia?

Answer: Assess for fluid overload because an elevated chloride level potentially includes an elevated sodium level. Signs and symptoms of fluid overload include agitation, edema, distended neck veins, elevated blood pressure, tachycardia, and dyspnea. Also monitor the acid–base balance closely. Symptoms of hyperchloremia mirror those of metabolic acidosis: confusion, Kussmaul's respirations, tachypnea, lethargy, and weakness.

QUICK LOOK AT THE CHAPTER AHEAD

Hypochloremia is defined as a serum chloride level of less than 98 mEq/L. It rarely occurs in the absence of other abnormalities. It usually occurs along with low serum sodium levels or an elevated serum bicarbonate level. Here we take a look at the causes associated with decreased intake of chloride, increased loss or decreased absorption, as well as manifestations and treatment for this condition.

22

Hypochloremia

TERMS
☐ Hypochloremia

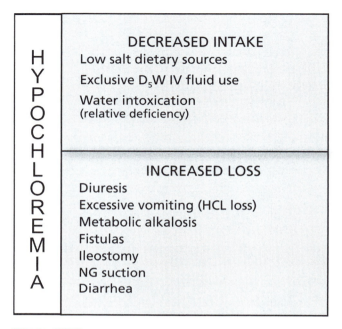

Figure 22-1 Decreased intake and increased loss.

CAUSES

Hypochloremia is defined as a serum chloride level of less than 98 mEq/L. It usually occurs along with low serum sodium levels or an elevated serum bicarbonate level (metabolic alkalosis).

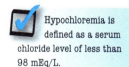

Hypochloremia is defined as a serum chloride level of less than 98 mEq/L.

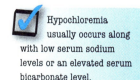

Hypochloremia usually occurs along with low serum sodium levels or an elevated serum bicarbonate level.

Decreased Intake

A low serum chloride level occurs when intake decreases through a low-salt diet. It also may occur with continuous administration of intravenous fluids without chloride, such as dextrose in water. In rare situations it may occur due to an extreme intake of free water.

Increased Loss and Decreased Absorption

An increase in chloride loss contributes to hypochloremia. Chloride is lost through the renal and gastrointestinal systems and through the skin with excessive sweating. Draining fistulas, ileostomies, or prolonged nasogastric suctioning without replacement of chloride can cause a hypochloremic state. Excessive vomiting and diarrhea are situations also related to chloride loss. When

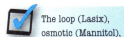 The loop (Lasix), osmotic (Mannitol), and thiazide (hydrochloro-thiazide) diuretics may also bring about a loss of chloride through a decreased absorption of water and electrolytes in the renal system.

hydrochloric acid is lost from the stomach, a situation of metabolic alkalosis can occur due to the fact that there is less competition for the bicarbonate ion with sodium. The loop (Lasix), osmotic (Mannitol), and thiazide (hydrochlorothiazide) diuretics may also bring about a loss of chloride through a decreased absorption of water and electrolytes in the renal system (Table 22-1). All losses contribute to decreased absorption.

Table 22-1 Causes of Hypochloremia

Metabolic alkalosis
    Fistulas
    Ileostomy
    Nasogastric suction
    Vomiting
    Diarrhea
    Medications (i.e., loop, osmotic, or potassium-sparing diuretics)
Hyponatremia
    Renal failure
    Syndrome of inappropriate antidiuretic hormone
    Congestive heart failure
    Burns
    Excessive sweating
    Medications (i.e., thiazide diuretics)
    Excessive intravenous intake of 5% dextrose in water

MANIFESTATIONS

Patients who suffer from hypochloremia manifest signs and symptoms associated with electrolyte imbalance, such as hyponatremia or hypokalemia (Table 22-2). The nerves become excitable, causing a hypertonicity of the muscles and a hyperactivity of the deep tendon reflexes. The patient may experience cramping, twitching, and eventual tetany of the muscles. Agitation and irritability also accompany these situations.

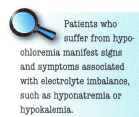

Patients who suffer from hypochloremia manifest signs and symptoms associated with electrolyte imbalance, such as hyponatremia or hypokalemia.

If a state of metabolic alkalosis occurs, the body will attempt to compensate by retaining carbon dioxide via the respiratory system. This is manifested by a slow respiratory rate.

TREATMENT

As with many electrolyte and acid–base disturbances, the treatment involves correction of the underlying cause. If a low-salt diet is the problem, then salt intake should be increased. Broth or juices such as tomato juice are helpful.

If too much chloride is lost via the gastrointestinal tract for various reasons, it may be replaced through intravenous fluids containing saline or oral supplements. Ammonium chloride may be given to increase the chloride level; however, this solution should not be given to patients with hepatic disease due to it being metabolized by the liver. Saline solution, not tap water, should be used for irrigation or flushing of any gastric tubes. If the hypochloremic condition is related to a low potassium, potassium chloride may be added to the intravenous solution or administered orally if the patient is allowed oral intake.

Table 22-2　Manifestations of Hypochloremia

Agitation
Irritability
Hypertonicity
Hyperactive reflexes
Cramping/twitching
Tetany

Question: What do I use to flush my patient's gastric tube?

Answer: Saline solution, not tap water, should be used for irrigation or flushing of any gastric tubes.

Question: What interventions are important for the patient with hypochloremia?

Answer: Monitor the patient's level of consciousness and cardiac rhythm. Assess electrolyte status frequently and observe for any acid–base imbalance. Carefully monitor the intake and output. If the patient is able to eat, offer oral supplements and foods high in chloride.

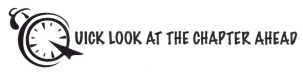

After potassium, magnesium is the second most prevalent cation in the intracellular fluid. The normal concentration of magnesium is 1.8 to 2.7 mEq/L. A well-balanced diet supplies the necessary daily requirement (300–350 mg) for the body. In this chapter we discuss the function, regulation, and balance of magnesium in the body.

23

Magnesium

TERMS
☐ **Magnesium**

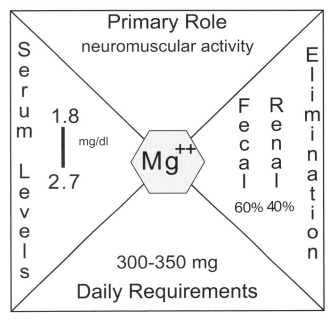

Figure 23-1 Primary role of magnesium.

FUNCTION

After potassium, **magnesium** is the second most prevalent cation in the intracellular fluid. The normal concentration of magnesium is 1.8 to 2.7 mEq/L with very little found in the extracellular fluid and approximately 60% located in the bones. Magnesium is similar to calcium in that it is found either ionized in a physiologically active form (approximately two-thirds) or bound, primarily with albumin, and considered physiologically inactive (one-third).

> The normal concentration of magnesium is 1.8 to 2.7 mEq/L with very little found in the extracellular fluid and approximately 60% located in the bones.

Magnesium functions within the cell, activating enzymes for protein synthesis and carbohydrate metabolism. It helps to carry sodium and potassium across the cell membrane in an effort to maintain electrolyte homeostasis. Magnesium has an effect on the parathyroid hormone, thereby influencing calcium levels. It also assists the body in the production of energy through the use and storage of adenosine triphosphate.

Magnesium acts as a transmitter of neuromuscular activity, particularly with the central nervous system, and helps with the contraction of heart muscle, keeping a steady rhythm. Magnesium assists the release of acetylcholine at the neuromuscular junction, directly affecting muscles.

REGULATION

A well-balanced diet supplies the necessary daily requirement (300–350 mg) for the body. Magnesium is found in various food sources such as seafood and meats; green leafy vegetables, which are rich in chlorophyll; dried beans; whole grains; peas; chocolate; and nuts. The body absorbs magnesium through the small intestine and excretes it via urine and feces.

Question: What types of foods provide a source of magnesium?

Answer: Dietary sources of magnesium are as follows:

- **Seafood and meats**
- **Vegetables, such as peas, green leafy vegetables, and broccoli**
- **Dried beans**
- **Whole grains**
- **Chocolate**
- **Nuts and seeds**
- **Peanut butter**
- **Oatmeal**
- **Potatoes and rice**
- **Raisins**
- **Fruit**
- **Milk**

BALANCE

A balance of magnesium is maintained in the body through absorption, excretion, or retention of the electrolyte via the gastrointestinal tract or renal system. If magnesium levels are low, the body absorbs more through the small intestine. When levels are too high, more is excreted by the kidneys through blockage of reabsorption in the proximal tubule and loop of Henle.

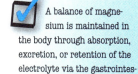

A balance of magnesium is maintained in the body through absorption, excretion, or retention of the electrolyte via the gastrointestinal tract or renal system.

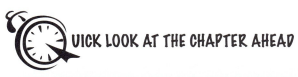

Hypermagnesemia occurs with a magnesium serum level greater than 2.7 mEq/L. The increased level occurs in the extracellular compartment and results from an increased intake or decreased excretion of magnesium. In this chapter we explain the causes, manifestations, and treatment for hypermagnesemia.

24

Hypermagnesemia

TERMS
☐ **Hypermagnesemia**

CAUSES

Hypermagnesemia is defined as a magnesium serum level greater than 2.7 mEq/L. The increased level occurs in the extracellular compartment and results from an increased intake or decreased excretion of magnesium. Though hypermagnesemia rarely occurs, an elevated level may result from an excessive intake of magnesium through magnesium-containing antacids or cathartics. It also may happen through an excessive administration of intravenous magnesium sulfate, particularly in the treatment of toxemia during pregnancy. Hypermagnesemia may also occur with the use of lithium (Figure 24-1).

A magnesium serum level greater than 2.7 mEq/L is considered to be hypermagnesemia.

Though hypermagnesemia rarely occurs, an elevated level may result from an excessive intake of magnesium through magnesium-containing antacids or cathartics.

The renal system is responsible for eliminating magnesium; therefore renal insufficiency or renal failure leads to elevated levels (Table 24-1).

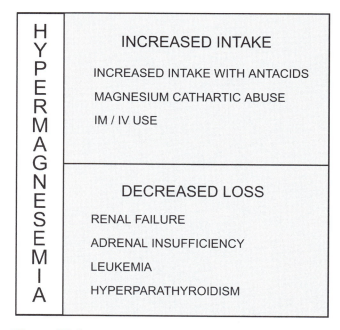

HYPERMAGNESEMIA	INCREASED INTAKE
	INCREASED INTAKE WITH ANTACIDS
	MAGNESIUM CATHARTIC ABUSE
	IM / IV USE
	DECREASED LOSS
	RENAL FAILURE
	ADRENAL INSUFFICIENCY
	LEUKEMIA
	HYPERPARATHYROIDISM

Figure 24-1 Increased intake and decreased loss.

Table 24-1 Causes of Hypermagnesemia

Medications
    Antacids
    Cathartics
    Magnesium sulfate
    Lithium
Dehydration
Hyperparathyroidism
Adrenal insufficiency
Leukemia
Renal failure

Severe dehydration secondary to diabetic ketoacidosis may cause a hemoconcentration of magnesium. A situation when magnesium may transiently elevate occurs during stages of hyperparathyroidism when magnesium shifts from the bone to the extracellular fluid. Adrenal insufficiency and leukemia are also known causes of hypermagnesemia.

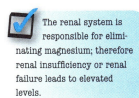
The renal system is responsible for eliminating magnesium; therefore renal insufficiency or renal failure leads to elevated levels.

MANIFESTATIONS

In states of hypermagnesemia the release of acetylcholine is decreased at the neuromuscular junction, depressing neuromuscular function. This causes central nervous system sedative effects such as decreased reflexes (Table 24-2). The patient may appear drowsy and lethargic. Diaphoresis and flushing occur. Muscles become weaker and flaccid as the serum magnesium level increases. The muscles of the respiratory system are especially affected, becoming depressed and resulting in slow shallow respirations and the potential for respiratory arrest. The excitability of the cardiac membrane also becomes depressed, and conduction decreases, resulting in bradycardia and hypotension. The possibility of cardiac dysrhythmias and possible cardiac arrest develop if the condition goes on unattended.

Too much magnesium especially affects the muscles of the respiratory system, which become depressed, resulting in slow shallow respirations and the potential of respiratory arrest.

Table 24-2 Manifestations of Hypermagnesemia

Warm flushed appearance
Diaphoresis
Nausea/vomiting/diarrhea
Drowsiness/lethargy
Weakness and flaccid muscles
Heart block and other dysrhythmias
Respiratory and cardiac arrest
Loss of deep tendon reflexes
Depressed respiratory system
    Slow respirations
    Shallow respirations
Hypotension
Bradycardia
Coma

TREATMENT

Treatment, as with many electrolyte imbalances, consists of correcting the underlying cause. Switching to a different antacid or stopping the use of laxatives may be necessary. Sodium inhibits renal tubular absorption of magnesium; therefore intravenous saline solutions are helpful. Increasing the fluid intake along with diuretics may also help to flush out the excess. If the patient has a renal condition, dialysis may be necessary. They should also be cautioned against using magnesium-containing antacids and laxatives.

Question: What interventions are important for the patient with hypermagnesemia?

Answer: Evaluate cognitive status, assessing for confusion. Monitor vital signs and cardiac status, assessing for hypotension, bradycardia, and potential dysrhythmias. Assess for slow and shallow respirations, which are signs of respiratory depression. Check for muscle weakness and deep tendon reflexes. Observe skin for a flushed and diaphoretic appearance. Monitor serum electrolyte status and fluid balance closely.

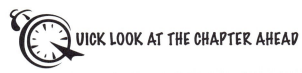

Hypomagnesemia is a condition that results in a magnesium blood level of < 1.5 mEq/L. Though magnesium deficiency is not frequently seen, a prevalence of low magnesium stores in the body suggests that dietary consumption of magnesium is below recommended levels. Many patients do not experience symptoms until the serum level reaches 1.0 mEq/L. Here we examine the causes, manifestations, and treatment of hypomagnesemia.

25

Hypomagnesemia

TERMS
☐ **Hypomagnesmia**

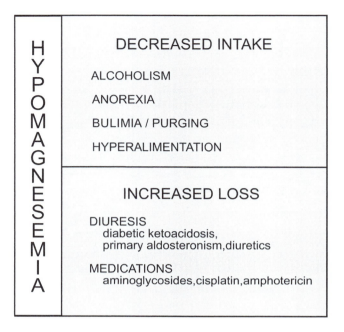

Figure 25-1 Decreased intake and increased loss.

CAUSES

Hypomagnesemia is a condition that results in a magnesium blood level of < 1.5 mEq/L, but many patients do not experience symptoms until the serum level reaches 1.0 mEq/L. It occurs more frequently than hypermagnesemia and results from decreased intake or absorption of magnesium or excessive loss. Other electrolyte imbalances such as hypokalemia, hypocalcemia, or metabolic acidosis may enhance the effects of low magnesium (Table 25-1).

 Hypomagnesemia is a condition that results in a magnesium blood level of <1.5 mEq/L, but many patients do not experience symptoms until the serum level reaches 1.0 mEq/L.

Decreased Intake

Hypomagnesemia is frequently seen with alcoholism because of a decreased dietary intake and, therefore, decreased absorption. Excessive

Table 25-1 Causes of Hypomagnesemia

Decreased Intake	Decreased Absorption	Excessive Loss
Alcoholism	Bulimia/purging	Diuresis
Anorexia	Laxatives	Diabetic ketoacidosis
Hyperalimentation	Chronic diarrhea	Hyperparathyroidism
	Fistula drainage	Primary aldosteronism
	Nasogastric drainage	Diuretics
		Burns/wounds
		Medications
		Cisplatin
		Digitalis
		Insulin
		Antibiotics
		Cyclosporine
		Amphotericin B
		Aminoglycosides

alcohol use also causes an increased loss through a high urine output or emesis. Anorexic patients suffer from multiple electrolyte imbalances, including hypomagnesemia. Patients who require long-term intravenous therapy during extended hospitalizations or hyperalimentation that are not supplemented with magnesium may suffer from hypomagnesemia.

Decreased Absorption

People who overuse laxatives or those who take part in the binging and purging syndrome of bulimia do not allow enough time for the absorption of magnesium through the small bowel. Patients who suffer from chronic diarrhea or fistula drainage lose magnesium through the fluids contained in the lower gastrointestinal tract. Patients with nasogastric suction may have decreased absorption in the intestine due to loss of magnesium from the upper gastrointestinal tract.

Excessive Loss

Magnesium is lost through the renal system and affects anyone suffering from excessive diuresis, such as that which accompanies diabetic ketoacidosis, hyperparathyroidism, or primary aldosteronism. Excessive or prolonged use of diuretics, particularly the more aggressive diuretics such as the thiazide or loop diuretics, results in an increased loss of fluid and therefore an increased loss and exchange of electrolytes, including magnesium. Patients suffering from serious burns or wounds also lose magnesium through the injured area. The use of certain antibiotics such as cyclosporine, amphotericin B, and aminoglycoside antibiotics may contribute to the loss of magnesium through increased urinary excretion. Cisplatin, used in chemotherapy, or digitalis and insulin are other commonly used drugs that affect the magnesium level.

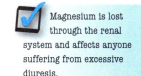
Magnesium is lost through the renal system and affects anyone suffering from excessive diuresis.

MANIFESTATIONS

Hypomagnesemia frequently occurs along with low potassium and calcium levels. This combined effect can result in cardiac and neurological manifestations (Table 25-2). The loss of magnesium affects the neuromuscular, central nervous, cardiovascular, and gastrointestinal systems. Symptoms may go unnoticed or may cause a life-threatening condition.

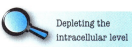
Depleting the intracellular level of magnesium leaves the cell weak, contributing to weakened skeletal muscles and hyperirritable nerves and muscles. Hypomagnesemia + hypokalemia + hypocalcemia = neuromuscular problems and cardiac dysrhythmias.

Table 25-2 Manifestations of Hypomagnesemia

Neuromuscular	Cardiac
Hyperirritable nerves and muscles	Prolonged PR and QT intervals
Altered level of consciousness	Prolonged QRS complex
Emotional lability/depression	Depressed ST segment
Tremors/twitching/spasticity	Flattened T with U wave
Hyperactive deep tendon reflexes	Premature ventricular contractions
Chvostek's sign	Supraventricular tachycardia
Trousseau's sign	Ventricular tachycardia
Nystagmus	Ventricular fibrillation
Seizures	Digitalis toxicity
Compromised respiratory system	Anorexia
	Nausea/vomiting
	Dysrhythmias
	Yellow-green vision

Neuromuscular Manifestations

As magnesium leaves the body, more magnesium flows out of the cell. Depleting the intracellular level of magnesium leaves the cell weak, contributing to weakened skeletal muscles and hyperirritable nerves and muscles. Compared with hypermagnesemia, where the muscles become weak, in hypomagnesemia the muscles become hyperactive, developing tremors, twitching, spasticity, and hyperactive deep tendon reflexes. Chvostek's sign (tapping the facial nerve, observing for facial twitching) and Trousseau's sign (compressing the upper arm, observing for carpal spasm) are positive. Nystagmus and seizures may occur. The respiratory muscles may also be affected, compromising breathing.

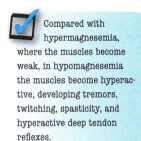

Compared with hypermagnesemia, where the muscles become weak, in hypomagnesemia the muscles become hyperactive, developing tremors, twitching, spasticity, and hyperactive deep tendon reflexes.

Central Nervous System Manifestations

Central nervous system irritability involves an altered level of consciousness, leading to confusion, personality change, depression, delusions, or hallucinations. Patients exhibit anxiety and irritability.

Cardiac Manifestations

When the magnesium level drops the activity of the enzyme that propels the potassium–sodium pump decreases, causing a decreased flow of potassium into the cell. The cardiac muscle becomes irritable and dysrhythmias develop. Specific segments of the electrocardiogram become prolonged, such as the PR interval, QRS complex, and QT interval, or depressed, such as the ST segment, allowing for the interference of irritable beats. Dangerous dysrhythmias can range from premature ventricular contractions to ventricular tachycardia and fibrillation. The risk of digitalis toxicity must not be overlooked. A decreased magnesium level increases the retention of digitalis. Combined with low potassium, the cardiac muscle could be in severe jeopardy.

Patients taking digitalis must be closely monitored for decreased magnesium levels. A decreased magnesium level increases the retention of digitalis. Combined with low potassium, the cardiac muscle could be in severe jeopardy.

Gastrointestinal Manifestations

Patients with hypomagnesemia suffer from difficulty swallowing (dysphagia). They tend to have bouts of nausea and vomiting and become anorexic. This leads to a poor dietary intake.

TREATMENT

If the patient is suffering from low potassium and magnesium, replacing the potassium does not relieve symptoms until the magnesium level is brought to normal first. This is an important concept to remember with patients taking digoxin and diuretics. If the situation is severe, the replacement of magnesium should be done intravenously. If the level is not too low, oral supplements (magnesium oxide) may be used. As with any electrolyte disturbance, discovering the underlying cause for the imbalance must be accomplished.

Question: What type of treatment should my patient receive for hypomagnesemia?

Answer: As with any electrolyte disturbance, discovering the underlying cause for the imbalance must be accomplished.

Question: What interventions are important for the patient with hypomagnesemia?

Answer: Assess level of consciousness for irritability, confusion, or delusions. Evaluate for muscle weakness, hyperirritable nerves and deep tendon reflexes, and the potential for seizures. Respiratory airway may be compromised by laryngeal stridor; therefore assess respiratory status frequently. Monitor cardiac status closely for dysrhythmias. Administer intravenous magnesium sulfate, if ordered, slowly and with an infusion pump. Keep calcium gluconate at the bedside in the event of too much magnesium replacement.

PART II · QUESTIONS

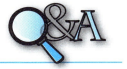

1. Two main systems for regulating water levels are
   (A) Low blood volume and sodium excretion
   (B) Osmoreceptors and the renal system
   (C) ADH and cellular dehydration
   (D) The thirst mechanism and ADH

2. Which of the following conditions is the result of too much fluid in the vascular compartment?
   (A) Edema
   (B) Hypervolemia
   (C) Hypovolemia
   (D) Hypernatremia

3. Which of the following would be a dangerous outcome of intracellular fluid overload?
   (A) Cerebral cellular rupture
   (B) Hypervolemia
   (C) Cellular dehydration
   (D) Congestive heart failure

4. Loss of body water along with a loss of sodium contributes to
   (A) Hypernatremia
   (B) Intracellular fluid overload
   (C) Fluid volume deficit
   (D) An increase in electrolytes

5. Which of the following is the *most* important cation in the extracellular fluid?
   (A) Potassium
   (B) Calcium
   (C) Chloride
   (D) Sodium

6. Hyperglycemia may cause which of the following conditions?
   (A) Hypercalcemia
   (B) Hypoosmolar hyponatremia
   (C) Hyperosmolar hyponatremia
   (D) Hypocalcemia

7. Potassium is primarily excreted from the body via
   (A) Cellular exchange
   (B) Feces
   (C) Urine
   (D) Breathing

8. A greater loss of water compared with salt or an acute gain of salt compared with water results in which of the following conditions?
   (A) Hyperkalemia
   (B) Hypernatremia
   (C) Hyponatremia
   (D) Hypokalemia

9. A way to move potassium back into the cell during critical states of hyperkalemia is
   (A) Diuretics
   (B) Insulin and glucose
   (C) Potassium supplement
   (D) Increased dietary intake of potassium

10. Calcium is primarily stored in the
   (A) Cells and fluid compartments
   (B) Cardiac and smooth muscle
   (C) Protein and small organic ions
   (D) Bones and teeth

11. High chloride levels occur in combination with excess _____ and decreased _____.
   (A) Sodium, bicarbonate
   (B) Potassium, calcium
   (C) Bicarbonate, sodium
   (D) Parathyroid hormone, sodium

12. Which of the following electrolytes is the second most prevalent cation in the intracellular fluid?

(A) Sodium

(B) Magnesium

(C) Calcium

(D) Chloride

13. Parathyroid hormone helps to activate calcium from bone and therefore is responsible for

(A) Hypernatremia

(B) Hypokalemia

(C) Hypercalcemia

(D) Hypocalcemia

14. Trousseau's and Chvostek's signs are tests reflective of

(A) Hypercalcemia

(B) Hypocalcemia

(C) Carpal spasm

(D) Decreased muscle excitability

PART II • ANSWERS AND RATIONALES

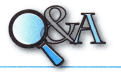

1. The correct answer is D.
   Rationale: Both thirst and ADH are sensitive to osmolality and extracellular fluid volume. The other choices play a role in water balance or are an outcome of too little fluid volume.

2. The correct answer is B.
   Rationale: Too much fluid in the vascular compartment is known as hypervolemia. Edema is associated with fluid overload in the interstitial space. Hypovolemia is too little fluid in the vascular compartment. Hypernatremia is too much sodium and a probable cause of hypervolemia.

3. The correct answer is A.
   Rationale: Cells can rupture from too much fluid. The cells in the brain are the most vulnerable to this. Hypervolemia is too much fluid in the vascular compartment. Cellular dehydration is the opposite of fluid overload. Congestive heart failure results from a weakened left ventricle, possibly from too much fluid in the vascular compartment, not fluid in the cells.

4. The correct answer is C.
   Rationale: When sodium is lost from the body, water follows, causing a deficit in fluid volume. Hypernatremia is a condition of too much sodium, not a loss. Intracellular fluid overload is the result of too much fluid in the cells. An increase in electrolytes is vague and unrelated to what the question is asking.

5. The correct answer is D.
   Rationale: Sodium is the most prevalent and important cation in the extracellular fluid (135–148 mEq/L). Potassium is the most important in the intracellular compartment. Calcium is predominately found in the bones and teeth. Chloride is an anion.

6. The correct answer is C.
Rationale: Increased glucose causes a hyperosmolar state. Water shifts to the area of increased glucose outside the cell, diluting the extracellular compartment. This causes a hyponatremia in a hyperosmolar state. Calcium does not play a role in this situation and answer B is not associated with hyperglycemia.

7. The correct answer is C.
Rationale: Potassium is primarily lost from the body via the renal system. Cellular exchange takes place during states of acidosis. Potassium is lost through feces, but only states of profuse diarrhea cause a decrease in potassium levels.

8. The correct answer is B.
Rationale: Hyponatremia is an excess of water compared with sodium. Hypo- and hyperkalemia refer to potassium.

9. The correct answer is B.
Rationale: The combination of insulin and glucose helps drive potassium back into the cell. Potassium supplements and an increased dietary intake only increase the potassium level, which is already elevated. Diuretics eliminate potassium through the renal system but do not assist in moving the ion back into the intracellular compartment.

10. The correct answer is D.
Rationale: Ninety-nine percent of calcium is located in the bones and teeth. The other 1% is found in the extracellular compartment, and more than one-third is bound to protein. Calcium functions in the contraction of cardiac and skeletal muscle.

11. The correct answer is A.
Rationale: Chloride loves to bind with sodium and works inversely with bicarbonate; therefore when sodium levels are high, chloride levels are also elevated and bicarbonate levels are decreased. Potassium is exchanged for chloride in conditions of hyperkalemia, with potassium elimination taking place while chloride is retained. Hyperparathyroidism caused by elevated parathyroid hormone levels may contribute to hyperchloremia, but sodium will not be decreased as suggested with answer D.

12. The correct answer is B.
Rationale: Magnesium is the second most prevalent cation in the intracellular fluid. Sodium is the most prevalent cation in the extracellular fluid. Calcium is a cation with somewhat equal concentrations in both the extracellular and intracellular fluid, and chloride is an anion prevalent in the extracellular fluid.

13. The correct answer is C.
Rationale: The parathyroid hormone helps activate calcium from bone, and when excess parathyroid hormone is produced it can be responsible for causing hypercalcemia.

14. The correct answer is B.
Rationale: Hypocalcemia generates neuromuscular irritability manifested by a positive Chvostek's or Trousseau's sign. Hypercalcemia causes a decrease in neuromuscular excitability. Carpal spasm, elicited by occluding the arterial blood flow to the hand for ~3 minutes, is the positive indicator for Trousseau's sign. A facial twitch when the facial nerve is tapped is indicative of a positive Chvostek's sign. As a reminder, these signs are also positive with patients experiencing hypomagnesemia.

III

Acid-Base

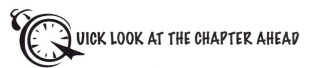

In this chapter we discuss the hydrogen ion and its relationship to pH. The regulation of pH through the buffering systems is also identified.

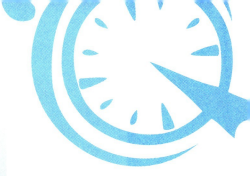

26

Acid-Base

TERMS
☐ **Hydrogen ion**

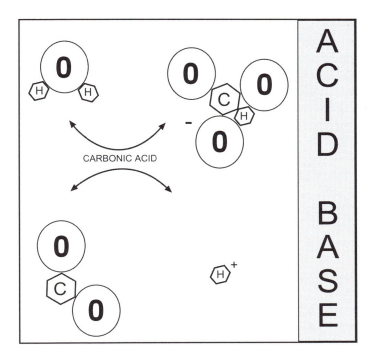

Figure 26-1 Acid–base.

UNDERSTANDING PH

The amount of acid or base in body fluid is reflected in the pH, the negative logarithm of the hydrogen ion (H^+). The **hydrogen ion** (acid) is needed for maintenance of cellular membranes and enzyme reactions, and minor alterations may affect metabolism and essential body functions. It travels in the body fluid as a volatile acid, carbonic acid (H_2CO_3). It breaks down into H^+ and HCO_3^-. The volatile gas, CO_2, is expelled through breathing, and the remaining part of the compound forms with other ions to make nonvolatile acids that are excreted in the urine. Nonvolatile acids such as the noncarbonic acids (hydrochloric, phosphoric, etc.) are buffered and then eliminated via the renal system, not the respiratory system.

Because acid–base balance is controlled primarily by the respiratory and renal systems, disorders affecting these systems affect the pH balance.

Many disease processes affecting the acid–base balance of the body may produce life-threatening alterations more damaging than the actual pathological condition.

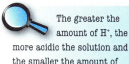

Many disease processes affecting the acid–base balance of the body may produce life-threatening alterations more damaging than the actual pathological condition.

The small concentration of H^+ in the bloodstream (0.0000001 mg/L or 10^{-7}) is indicated as pH 7.0. An important concept to remember is that the greater the amount of H^+, the more acidic the solution and the smaller the amount of H^+, the more basic or alkaline the solution. Because pH is based on a negative

The greater the amount of H^+, the more acidic the solution and the smaller the amount of H^+, the more basic or alkaline the solution.

logarithm, the value lowers with higher H^+ concentrations and raises with lower H^+ concentrations; therefore a low pH value equals an acidic solution and a high pH value indicates the solution is alkaline (Figure 26-2). The normal range for arterial blood is a pH level between 7.35 and 7.45. Death generally results if the levels fall below 6.9 or above 7.8.

REGULATION OF PH

The metabolic breakdown of proteins, carbohydrates, and fats produces hydrogen ions that can combine to form acids. Three systems help to maintain acid–base homeostasis: buffers, the respiratory system, and the renal system. Buffers are chemicals that

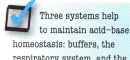

Three systems help to maintain acid–base homeostasis: buffers, the respiratory system, and the renal system.

$\downarrow$ pH = $\uparrow$ H^+ concentration = Acidosis

$\uparrow$ pH = $\downarrow$ H^+ concentration = Alkalosis

Figure 26-2 pH value and acid–base.

combine with an acid or base to weaken or neutralize it. Buffering is an immediate reaction to counteract the extreme changes in pH until other regulatory systems take over to manage the situation (see Chapter 27).

The respiratory system expels carbon dioxide as a method for maintaining acid–base balance. Hypoventilation allows for the retention of carbonic acid, and hyperventilation helps to expel the acid. Both are compensatory mechanisms that can act immediately to correct an acid–base imbalance (see Chapter 29).

The renal system is the slowest of the three systems to respond to an acid–base imbalance. Taking hours to days, it responds by excreting or reabsorbing the acid or base, whichever is required for regaining balance (see Chapter 28).

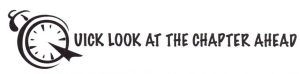

Metabolic regulation of the body's pH is controlled by proteins, carbonic acid–bicarbonate, phosphates, and the plasma potassium–hydrogen exchange. Some work outside the cell, some inside the cell, and others inside and outside the cell.

27

pH Regulation Through Buffering Systems

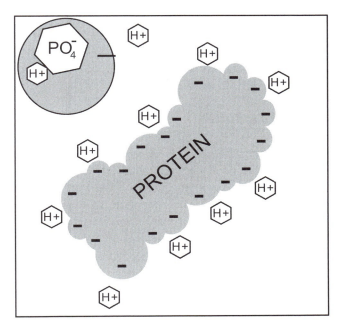

Figure 27-1 Protein.

BUFFERING SYSTEMS

Proteins, carbonic acid–bicarbonate, phosphates, and the plasma potassium–hydrogen exchange control the metabolic regulation of the body's pH, either by working outside the cell, inside the cell, or both inside and outside the cell. The protein and bicarbonate buffering systems are immediately available and the most effective in maintaining the proper body pH.

Protein Buffers

Proteins are the most plentiful buffering system, with a negative charge to buffer the hydrogen ion (H^+) and release or bind with it. Therefore proteins have the ability to function as an acid or base. Though proteins

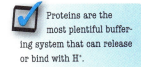
Proteins are the most plentiful buffering system that can release or bind with H^+.

exist inside and outside the cell, most are primarily located inside the cell, making this an intracellular buffering mechanism. H^+ and CO_2 diffuse across the cell membrane to bind with proteins inside the cell, whereas albumin and plasma globulins act as the primary protein buffers in the vascular compartment.

Carbonic Acid–Bicarbonate

This buffering system is the largest in the extracellular fluid, particularly plasma and interstitial fluid. Carbonic acid (H_2CO_3) and bicarbonate (HCO_3^-) are the major players working with the respiratory and renal systems. Carbon dioxide and water combine to form carbonic acid, $CO_2 + H_2O = H_2CO_3$, in the presence of the enzyme carbonic anhydrase, which catalyzes the reaction. As long as the rate of carbon dioxide being produced equals the rate in which it is expelled, H^+ concentration does not change. If there is an excess of H^+, the lungs can decrease the amount of carbonic acid through increased respirations, blowing off the CO_2 and leaving H_2O.

In the kidney Na^+ is reabsorbed into the tubular cell and H^+ is secreted into the tubular fluid. In acidotic states the renal system works by secreting excess H^+ to combine with bicarbonate (HCO_3^-), resulting in CO_2 and H_2O. The water is eliminated via urine, and the CO_2 travels to the tubular cell. With the help of the enzyme carbonic anhydrase, the CO_2 combines with H_2O in the tubular cell to make a new HCO_3^- and a free H^+. The HCO_3^- is then reabsorbed into the blood to combine with Na^+ and the lone H^+ starts another cycle in the tubular fluid.

If the situation is reversed, a state of alkalosis with a decreased number of H^+, the carbonic acid releases H^+ to help decrease the pH to normal. The respiratory system also tries to slow respirations in an attempt to retain CO_2. To maintain a normal pH of 7.40 the bicarbonate-to-carbonic acid ratio must be kept at 20:1. The respiratory and renal system work well together to keep this ratio. The respiratory system can work quickly to expel CO_2 and the renal system, though slower, easily reabsorbs or regenerates bicarbonate.

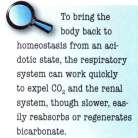 To bring the body back to homeostasis from an acidotic state, the respiratory system can work quickly to expel CO_2 and the renal system, though slower, easily reabsorbs or regenerates bicarbonate.

Phosphate Buffers

The phosphate buffering system acts much like the carbonic acid–bicarbonate system. Phosphates are highly concentrated in the intracellular fluid. Some of the phosphates act as weak acids to buffer stronger bases, and some act as a weak base to buffer a stronger acid. Buffering takes place predominately in the renal tubules where the greatest concentration of phosphates exists. The phosphate buffering system attempts to bring the pH back to normal by moving the H^+ from the plasma to the urine and eliminating the acid through urine.

Potassium–Hydrogen Exchange

These two positively charged ions move interchangeably in and out of the cell, depending on excess. When there is an excess of H^+ in the extracellular fluid, H^+ moves inside the cell for buffering and, in exchange, K^+ moves into the extracellular fluid. Therefore it is important to note that changes in potassium levels can affect the acid–base balance in the body, as can a state of acidosis affect the potassium level.

Changes in potassium levels can affect the acid–base balance in the body, as can a state of acidosis affect the potassium level.

The kidneys are effective in acid–base balance because they permanently remove the hydrogen ion from the body. Though efficient, with the ability to last longer than other buffers, the renal system takes days to become completely effective when regulating pH. In this chapter we look at the different chemical combinations the renal system uses to regulate an acid–base imbalance.

28

Renal Regulation

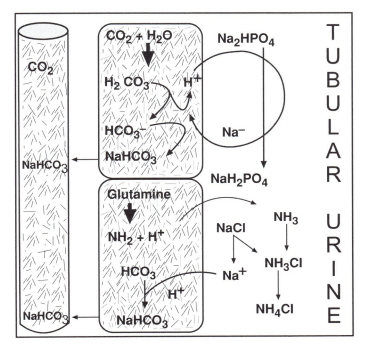

Figure 28-1 Tubular urine.

The kidneys are effective in acid–base balance because they permanently remove H^+ from the body. They also reabsorb acids or bases and produce bicarbonate ions. If the pH decreases, indicating a state of acidosis, the kidneys conserve or make new bicarbonate and excrete an acidic urine. Conversely, if the pH rises, indicating a state of alkalosis, the kidneys reabsorb the H^+ and excrete a more alkaline urine. Unlike the respiratory system, which can affect the pH in minutes, the renal processes are slow, taking hours to days to effectively regulate the pH; however, the effects of this system can last longer than other systems.

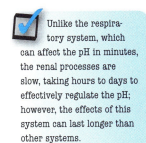

Unlike the respiratory system, which can affect the pH in minutes, the renal processes are slow, taking hours to days to effectively regulate the pH; however, the effects of this system can last longer than other systems.

HYDROGEN AND BICARBONATE

In the proximal tubule H^+ is secreted into the fluid to combine with HCO_3^-. This combination, carbonic acid–H_2CO_3, then forms CO_2 and H_2O. The H_2O is eliminated with the urine, and the CO_2 diffuses into the tubular cell. The CO_2 through a carbonic anhydrase-mediated reaction helps to create HCO_3^- and H^+ and the cycle continues.

TUBULAR SYSTEM

The urine pH is maintained between 4.5 and 8.0. To keep too many free H^+ from making the urine overly acidic and therefore too caustic to the urinary tract, phosphate and ammonia buffering systems exist. The phosphate system tends to work best with high concentrations of hydrogen. This is because phosphate is poorly reabsorbed and remains concentrated in the tubules, allowing for more hydrogen to be gathered for buffering. Ammonia ions, NH_3, once secreted into the tubular fluid combine with H^+ to make ammonium NH_4^+. Ammonium ions are effective buffers because they are lipid soluble and cannot cross from the tubular fluid back into the blood. The ammonium then combines with Cl^-, forming ammonium chloride (NH_4Cl), and is excreted in the urine (Figure 28-2). This system takes several days to generate sufficient amounts of ammonia to adequately buffer the acid.

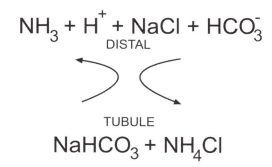

Figure 28-2 Distal tubule.

HYDROGEN AND POTASSIUM

Hydrogen is exchanged for potassium in the cell as potassium leaves the cell and enters the plasma during a state of acidosis. Consequently, the amount of hydrogen ions decreases while the potassium level increases in the extracellular fluid. Alkalosis has the opposite effect by decreasing potassium levels.

Acid Exchange

In a state of acidosis with excess carbonic acid, the kidneys help to maintain balance within the system by excreting other acids in an attempt to keep the pH from becoming exceedingly abnormal. If a lack of carbonic acid exists, then the kidneys work to retain other metabolic acids to maintain a balanced pH. This compensatory response takes several days to become completely efficient.

The respiratory system provides a quick response to an acid–base imbalance through control of the partial pressure of carbon dioxide ($PaCO_2$) in the arterial blood. In this chapter we examine the effects of respiratory regulation in an acid–base imbalance and how it controls acid through hyper- and hypoventilation.

29

Respiratory Regulation

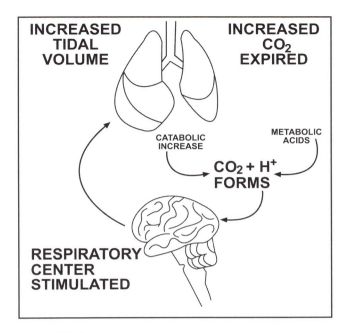

Figure 29-1 Increased tidal volume.

The respiratory system provides a quick response to an acid–base imbalance through control of the partial pressure of carbon dioxide ($PaCO_2$) in the arterial blood. When 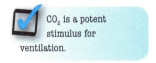 levels are elevated, CO_2 is a potent stimulus for ventilation. Carried by the red blood cell, carbon dioxide readily diffuses across the blood–brain barrier, reacting with H_2O to form H_2CO_3, which in turn splits into HCO_3 and H^+.

It is H^+ that is responsible for stimulating the respiratory drive. Increased amounts of H^+ cause an increase in respirations, and a decreased amount of H^+ results in decreased respirations. As ventilation increases CO_2 is blown off, leaving a decreased amount of carbon dioxide available to bond with H_2O. If acid is required for balancing the pH, a decreased respiratory rate helps to retain CO_2.

The body compensates with the various forms of nonvolatile acid to maintain proper pH balance. In situations of inadequate oxygen delivery, lactic acid develops from the anaerobic metabolism of glucose. If a heavy

CO_2 is a potent stimulus for ventilation.

load of lactic acid is circulating in the blood-stream, the body attempts to balance this increased acid-to-base ratio by eliminating CO_2 through an increased respiratory rate. The only way the respiratory system can remove acids is through the elimination of CO_2 from carbonic acid. It cannot remove other acids.

It is important to note that compensating for the increased acid does not correct the problem. If another acid is prevalent in the body, the respiratory system eliminates the CO_2 in an attempt to compensate for the low pH and to keep the pH from becoming dangerously low. The level of the particular acid initially responsible for the low pH, however, remains unchanged until other buffering mechanisms can remove the offending acid.

The respiratory system responds immediately to shifts in pH balance with hypoventilation for retention of CO_2 or hyperventilation to deplete CO_2. Though the response is rapid, there is a lag time before HCO_3 can reach adequate levels. Generally, the respiratory system reaches its maximum response in 12–24 hours. Also, the body can maintain a changed respiratory rate for only a limited amount of time before fatiguing.

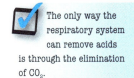

The only way the respiratory system can remove acids is through the elimination of CO_2.

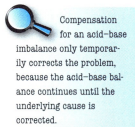

Compensation for an acid–base imbalance only temporarily corrects the problem, because the acid–base balance continues until the underlying cause is corrected.

In a state of acidosis the respiratory system attempts to decrease the increased acid through hyperventilation. In a state of alkalosis the respiratory system decreases the increased base through hypoventilation.

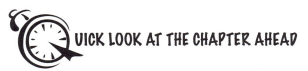

QUICK LOOK AT THE CHAPTER AHEAD

Metabolic acidosis results from a deficiency in HCO_3 (< 23 mEq/L) or an excess of noncarbonic acids. In metabolic acidosis the pH falls below 7.35. In this chapter we discuss the causes of metabolic acidosis and the manifestations of the condition and treatment.

30

Metabolic Acidosis

TERMS
☐ **Kussmaul respirations**

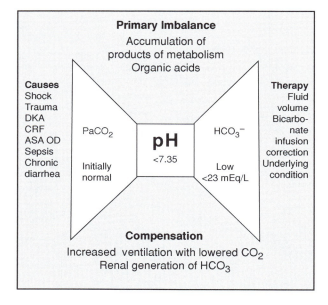

Figure 30-1 Primary imbalance.

CAUSES

Metabolic acidosis is the result of a deficiency in HCO_3 (< 23 mEq/L) or of an excess of noncarbonic acids. The pH is below 7.35 in metabolic acidosis.

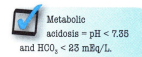

Metabolic acidosis = pH < 7.35 and HCO_3 < 23 mEq/L.

Bicarbonate Deficit

A bicarbonate deficit can occur through the loss of excessive intestinal secretions such as diarrhea, suction, or fistulas. A loss of HCO_3 can also occur through the renal system. Such conditions have the potential to cause a metabolic acidosis.

Excess Acid

Metabolic acidosis that results from increased acid levels can occur in situations involving an accumulation of lactic acid as in shock or cardiac arrest when anaerobic metabolism occurs due to insufficient oxygenation. Ketoacidosis can also result in metabolic acidosis, particularly with uncontrolled diabetes mellitus but also with excessive alcohol consumption, starvation, or ketogenic weight loss diets. Ingestion of methanol, ethylene glycol, or

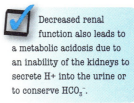 Decreased renal function also leads to a metabolic acidosis due to an inability of the kidneys to secrete H+ into the urine or to conserve HCO_3^-.

acetylsalicylic acid can produce extreme situations of metabolic acidosis and possible death. Decreased renal function also leads to a metabolic acidosis due to an inability of the kidneys to secrete H^+ into the urine or to conserve HCO_3^-. This frequently occurs in the elderly as renal function decreases and the kidneys cannot eliminate an increased amount of acid that has accumulated or been ingested.

Uncontrolled diabetes mellitus, excessive alcohol consumption, starvation, or ketogenic weight loss diets can result in ketoacidosis, which contributes to metabolic acidosis.

Hyperchloremic Acidosis

Hyperchloremic acidosis occurs with overtreatment of chloride-type medications, intravenous and hyperalimentation solutions, or increased absorption by the kidneys. Because HCO_3^- and Cl^- are both anions, the HCO_3^- concentration decreases when an excess of Cl^- are available. Ammonium chloride breaks down into NH_4^+ and Cl^-, allowing the ammonium ion to be converted to urea in the liver. This frees the Cl^-, allowing it to bind with available H^+. The combination forms hydrochloric acid, resulting in a situation of bicarbonate deficit and increased acid.

Anion Gap

Evaluation of the anion gap is helpful in determining the condition responsible for metabolic acidosis (Figure 30-2). The anion gap is used to identify the anions that are not measured. Conditions that result in a metabolic acidosis from excess acid create an increased anion gap. Normally, the sum of the cations is approximately equal to the sum of anions in the extracellular fluid. Sodium is the most plentiful cation in the extracellular fluid, and HCO_3^- and Cl^- are the most plentiful anions, with sodium usually outnumbering the bicarbonate and chloride ions. Therefore to

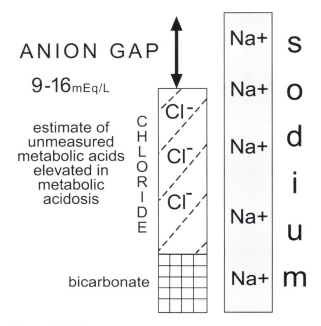

Figure 30-2 Anion gap.

determine the anion gap the bicarbonate and chloride results are added together and subtracted from sodium: $Na^+ - (HCO_3^- + CL^-)$. A normal anion gap is 9–6 mEq/L.

MANIFESTATIONS

A normal HCO_3^- level is 23–27 mEq/L. When the pH falls below 7.35 and the HCO_3^- level drops below 23 mEq/L, a metabolic acidosis exists. Metabolic acidosis results secondary to an existing problem. Therefore the characteristics of that particular disease process are manifested along with the acidosis. Frequently, patients in metabolic acidosis complain of headache, malaise, weakness, or fatigue (Table 30-1). Anorexia, nausea, and vomiting may accompany the other symptoms. The sympathetic nervous system, responsible for vasoconstriction, loses its control over the skin vessels, allowing them to dilate and make the skin warm and flushed. Cellular membrane excitability becomes depressed, and as the

Table 30-1 Manifestations of Metabolic Acidosis

Neurological	Cardiac
Headache	Decreased cardiac contractility
Malaise	Decreased cardiac output
Weakness	Dysrhythmias
Fatigue	Shock
Stupor/coma	
Sympathetic Nervous System	Respiratory
Vasodilation	Kussmaul respirations
Warm, flushed skin	
Gastrointestinal	Hyperkalemia
Nausea/vomiting	
Anorexia	

condition worsens the level of consciousness decreases to a stupor and eventual coma.

Cardiac contractility and output decrease and dysrhythmias develop as the pH continues to fall. Lactic acidosis begins to develop as ventricular function decreases and a shock state occurs. Acute metabolic acidosis is accompanied by respiratory compensation. The patient develops **Kussmaul respirations**, a breathing pattern of deep rapid respirations, in an attempt to eliminate acid via exhalation of CO_2.

Patients with chronic metabolic acidosis, such as that which accompanies renal failure, do not manifest all of the signs and symptoms as mentioned above because of the body's ability to compensate over time. In chronic renal failure the problem of acidosis affects the skeletal system with the release of calcium and phosphate for buffering excess H^+.

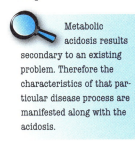

Metabolic acidosis results secondary to an existing problem. Therefore the characteristics of that particular disease process are manifested along with the acidosis.

TREATMENT

Supplemental HCO_3^- may be helpful, but not for conditions resulting in an increased ion gap. An example of this is a situation of lactic acidosis that occurs with cardiac arrest. This type of acidosis is often the result of inadequate oxygen perfusion. Adding more sodium bicarbonate to this scenario does not eliminate the oxygen problem and can cause hypernatremia and a state of hyperosmolality. It may also contribute to a decreased release of oxygen from the hemoglobin molecule, further complicating the lack of oxygen perfusion. The best treatment for metabolic acidosis is correcting the underlying problem and restoring fluid and electrolyte loss.

Question: **Many conditions can cause metabolic acidosis. What is the best treatment to help this condition?**

Answer: The best treatment for metabolic acidosis is correcting the underlying problem and restoring fluid and electrolyte loss.

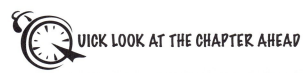 **QUICK LOOK AT THE CHAPTER AHEAD**

Metabolic alkalosis occurs when the bicarbonate level rises above 27 mEq/L and the pH above 7.45. It may result from an excess of HCO_3^-, a deficit of acid, or a combination of both. Here we discuss the causes, manifestations, and treatment of metabolic alkalosis.

31

Metabolic Alkalosis

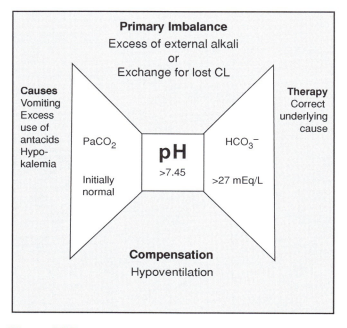

Figure 31-1 Primary imbalance.

CAUSES

Metabolic alkalosis occurs when the bicarbonate level rises above 27 mEq/L and the pH above 7.45. It may result from an excess of HCO_3^-, a deficit of acid, or a combination of both. The body's production and reabsorption of bicarbonate are usually maintained in a balance so that alkalosis does not occur. However, an intake of excess bicarbonate through antacids or overuse of bicarbonate products such as parenteral solutions containing lactate, hyperalimentation, or citrate with blood transfusions can increase the bicarbonate level above 27 mEq/L and move the pH above 7.45.

Another possible cause is the removal of H^+ and Cl^- from the stomach through emesis

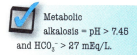
Metabolic alkalosis = pH > 7.45 and HCO_3^- > 27 mEq/L.

Metabolic alkalosis occurs when the body loses too much acid, such as severe situations of gastric suction, vomiting, binge–purge, or use of diuretics. Metabolic alkalosis can also occur when too much base is absorbed, such as with overuse of antacids or products containing bicarbonate.

or gastric suction, resulting in an excess of base. In situations where K^+ is lost, such as through the use of diuretics or metabolic disorders, H^+ excretion is increased as the kidneys work to conserve K^+. The body also shifts the hydrogen ion into the cell during conditions of hypokalemia and increases renal excretion of acid, contributing to or causing metabolic alkalosis.

MANIFESTATIONS

Patients with metabolic alkalosis resulting from a loss of body fluids through gastric suction, vomiting, binge–purge syndrome, or excessive diuretic use also manifest signs of volume depletion, such as postural hypotension or hypokalemia. When the condition is acute mental confusion occurs along with hyperactive reflexes, tingling, and tetany, leading to possible seizures. Respiratory failure, dysrhythmias, and eventual coma are manifestations of severe metabolic alkalosis with a pH > 7.55 (Table 31-1).

Respiratory failure, dysrhythmias, and eventual coma are manifestations of severe metabolic alkalosis with a pH > 7.55.

Table 31-1 Manifestations of Metabolic Alkalosis

Volume Depletion
    Postural hypotension
    Hypokalemia
Neurological
    Acute onset
        Mental confusion
        Hyperactive reflexes
        Tingling
        Tetany
        Seizures
pH > 7.55
    Respiratory failure
    Cardiac dysrhythmias
    Coma

TREATMENT

The compensatory mechanism for metabolic alkalosis is hypoventilation. By retaining CO_2 the body is increasing the acid content of the blood, because CO_2 combines with H_2O to make carbonic acid. Treatment is again aimed at the underlying cause of the problem. If a chloride or potassium deficit exists, correcting the reason for the loss and supplementing with potassium chloride help to correct the problem. Patients suffering from an extracellular fluid loss are given replacement with normal or one-half normal saline solution.

Question: **How does the body normally respond to a state of metabolic alkalosis?**

Answer: **The body responds by retaining acid (CO_2) through hypoventilation. The best treatment, however, is aimed at correcting the underlying cause of the problem.**

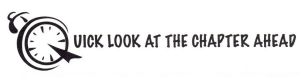
Respiratory acidosis occurs when the pH value decreases below 7.35 and the PCO$_2$ level rises above 45 mm Hg. Causes may be acute or chronic. In this chapter we describe the conditions that may cause respiratory acidosis, the manifestations, and the treatment, which is aimed at relieving the hypoxia and hypercapnia.

32

Respiratory Acidosis

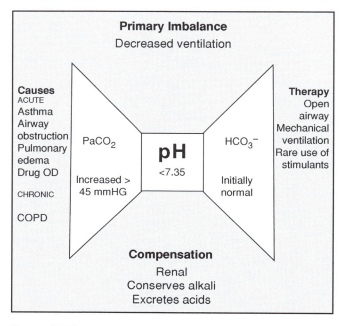

Figure 32-1 Primary imbalance.

CAUSES

Respiratory acidosis occurs when the pH value decreases below 7.35 and the PCO_2 level rises above 45 mm Hg from hypoventilation. Alveolar ventilation becomes impaired, caus-

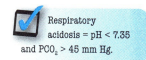

Respiratory acidosis = pH < 7.35 and PCO_2 > 45 mm Hg.

ing an increase in carbon dioxide and carbonic acid. The carbonic acid dissociates, allowing for free H^+, which contributes to the drop in pH. Acute and chronic conditions may be responsible.

Acute Respiratory Acidosis

Acute respiratory acidosis may be caused by trauma that causes chest injury and impairs the respiratory system. A bronchial asthma attack, a sudden onset of pulmonary edema, drug overdose, airway obstruction, or head trauma causing a brainstem injury may also lead to difficulty breathing and the subsequent development of acidosis. The elderly have the potential to succumb to respiratory depression and therefore respiratory acidosis. As one ages the ability to clear drugs efficiently through the renal system is decreased; therefore taking medications, such as barbiturates, can cause a respiratory depression due to the decreased renal clearance.

Chronic Respiratory Acidosis

In long-term lung diseases, such as emphysema or chronic obstructive lung disease, areas of the respiratory system are permanently compromised in their ability to exchange CO_2 and O_2. Because such lung diseases are conditions that occur over time, the body adjusts to a permanently high carbon dioxide level, known as hypercapnia, and the hypoxemia or respiratory acidosis is the stimulus for respiration. In addition, the renal system continues to work to secrete H^+ and reabsorb HCO_3^- as an attempt at compensation.

Patients with chronic respiratory disease can suffer from acute respiratory acidosis if O_2 is administered at a rate to suppress the stimulus for respirations. The patient's medullary respiratory center becomes accustomed to the elevated PCO_2 levels. The respiratory drive then comes from the O_2 content in the blood. If the O_2 level is increased beyond the point of its normal stimulus, the patient's rate and depth of respiration becomes suppressed and the CO_2 content increases.

> Lung diseases that occur over time allow the body to adjust to a permanently high carbon dioxide level, known as hypercapnia, and the hypoxemia or respiratory acidosis becomes the stimulus for respiration.

Patients with chronic respiratory disease can suffer from acute respiratory acidosis if O_2 is administered at a rate to suppress the stimulus for respirations.

MANIFESTATIONS

Carbon dioxide readily diffuses across the blood–brain barrier, causing neurological manifestations in the patient with respiratory acidosis (Table 32-1). Headache occurs because the blood vessels in the brain

Table 32-1 Manifestations of Respiratory Acidosis

Neurological	Cardiac
Headache	Tachycardia
Blurred vision	Peripheral vasodilation
Tremors	
Muscle twitching	Respiratory
Vertigo	Initial hyperventilation
Irritability	Eventual hypoventilation
Disorientation	
Lethargy	
Coma	

dilate, which allows for more fluid to enter the vessel and increases the cerebrospinal fluid pressure. Other neurological manifestations, such as blurred vision, tremors and muscle twitching, vertigo, irritability, and disorientation, occur secondary to the decreased pH of the cerebrospinal and interstitial fluids. Mild situations of acidosis result in flushed warm skin and weakness. In severe cases lethargy progresses to coma if the pH remains unchanged. A decreased intracellular pH affects the cardiac cells, causing tachycardia and other dysrhythmias. Peripheral vasodilation may occur, resulting in hypotension that may exacerbate the occurrence of dysrhythmias.

TREATMENT

Treatment is aimed at relieving the hypoxia and hypercapnia. If necessary, an airway must be established. Mechanical ventilation may be necessary for respiratory or neurological failure. The kidneys cannot excrete carbonic acid but can excrete metabolic acids and will do so in an attempt to compensate the pH. They will also make and reabsorb bicarbonate. The renal compensatory mechanism takes at least 24 hours to initiate and days to reach maximal effectiveness.

Respiratory alkalosis is associated with a carbonic acid deficit leading to a pH level greater than 7.45 and a CO_2 blood content of less than 7.35 mm Hg. Respiratory alkalosis secondary to hyperventilation may be intentional, as with mechanical ventilation, or accidental, as with a panic attack. In this chapter we examine the causes, manifestations, and treatment of respiratory alkalosis.

33

Respiratory Alkalosis

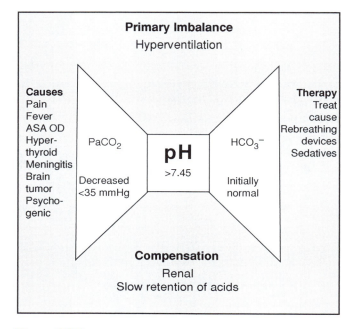

┌───┐
│ **Primary Imbalance** │
│ Hyperventilation │
│ │
│ **Causes**   **Therapy** │
│ Pain   Treat │
│ Fever   cause │
│ ASA OD   Rebreathing │
│ Hyper- $PaCO_2$ HCO_3^- devices │
│ thyroid   **pH**   Sedatives │
│ Meningitis   >7.45 │
│ Brain   Decreased   Initially │
│ tumor   <35 mmHg   normal │
│ Psycho- │
│ genic │
│ │
│ **Compensation** │
│ Renal │
│ Slow retention of acids │
└───┘

Figure 33-1 Respiratory alkalosis.

CAUSES

Respiratory alkalosis is the result of alveolar hyperventilation and a loss of carbon dioxide (hypocapnia) faster than the body can replace it. It is associated with a carbonic

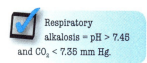

Respiratory alkalosis = pH > 7.45 and CO_2 < 7.35 mm Hg.

acid deficit that leads to a pH > 7.45 and a CO_2 blood content of less than 7.35 mm Hg. Respiratory alkalosis occurs secondary to hyperventilation when too much carbonic acid is expelled during expiration. The respirations are rapid and deep in hyperventilation. Panic attacks that result from high anxiety are a common cause of respiratory alkalosis. A less common cause is gram-negative septicemia, which triggers the respiratory center in the brainstem to increase respirations to the point of hyperventilation. Other causes are fever or oxygen deprivation, such as that triggered in high altitudes. The early stages of salicylate toxicity also stimulate the medullary respiratory center of the brainstem to hyperventilate. An intentional cause for hyperventilation is through anesthesia or mechanical ventilation.

MANIFESTATIONS

Symptoms of respiratory alkalosis are related to central nervous system irritability (Table 33-1). Neuromuscular excitability is a manifestation of decreased calcium levels secondary to the binding of calcium to protein. This causes numbness and tingling (paresthesias) around the mouth, fingers, and toes. Positive Chvostek's and Trousseau's signs may be present. Cramps or carpopedal spasms may also be present. CO_2 easily crosses the blood–brain barrier, causing vasoconstriction and a decreased cerebral blood flow. This results in lightheadedness and dizziness. Sweating, palpitation, panic, or air hunger may also be present.

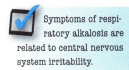

Symptoms of respiratory alkalosis are related to central nervous system irritability.

TREATMENT

Treating the underlying cause and increasing the CO_2 level are of primary importance. Recognizing the initial problem is helpful because many conditions are short-lived, such as panic attacks. Allowing one to rebreathe CO_2, such as when blowing into a paper bag, is helpful for anxiety-induced alkalosis. The kidneys attempt to retain H^+. However, this compensatory response takes several days.

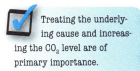

Treating the underlying cause and increasing the CO_2 level are of primary importance.

Table 33-1 Manifestations of Respiratory Alkalosis

Muscular Excitability
    Numbness/tingling
    Cramps/carpopedal spasms
    Decreased cerebral flood flow (i.e., lightheadedness, dizziness)
Sweating
Palpitation
Panic
Air Hunger

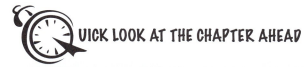
Compensation is the body's attempt to bring the acid–base imbalance back to normal. When compensating an acid-base disturbance, the system not responsible for the imbalance attempts to bring the blood pH back to normal. Compensation, however, is not correction. Unless the underlying condition is rectified, the imbalance is not corrected. In this chapter we discuss the compensatory mechanisms for acid–base disturbances.

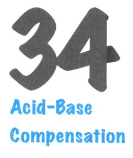

Acid-Base Compensation

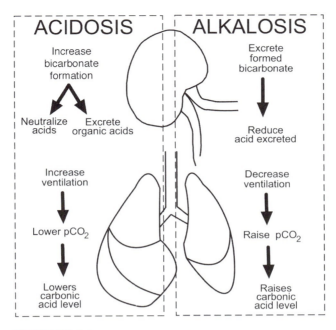

Figure 34-1 Acidosis and alkalosis.

As mentioned previously, the body has built-in mechanisms to compensate for acid–base imbalances. Compensation, however, is not correction. It is the body's attempt to bring the imbalance back to normal. Unless the underlying condition is rectified, the imbal-

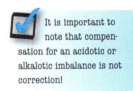

It is important to note that compensation for an acidotic or alkalotic imbalance is not correction!

ance is not corrected. When compensating an acid-base disturbance, the system not responsible for the imbalance attempts to bring the blood pH back to normal.

METABOLIC ACIDOSIS

In metabolic acidosis the respiratory system attempts to compensate by increasing the rate and depth of respirations through hyperventilation. When the pH drops below normal, the peripheral chemoreceptors stimulate the respiratory system in the brainstem. This increases the rate and depth of respirations in an attempt to blow off CO_2 and therefore to lower the carbonic acid blood level. By lowering the carbonic acid level, there is less acid in the blood for the bicarbonate to buffer, helping to raise the bicarbonate levels. The arterial blood gases in a patient with a compensated metabolic acidosis show a slightly low or normal pH level of 7.35–7.40, a decreased HCO_3 (initial problem) level less than 23 mEq/L, and a decreased PCO_2 (compensatory response) less than 35 mm Hg.

In metabolic acidosis the respiratory system attempts to compensate by increasing the rate and depth of respirations through hyperventilation. Blowing off CO_2 eliminates excess acid from the body, allowing for more bicarbonate to buffer the remaining acid.

METABOLIC ALKALOSIS

In metabolic alkalosis the respiratory system again attempts to compensate, and this time it decreases its rate and depth of respirations through hypoventilation. Through decreased and shallow respirations, CO_2 is retained and the carbonic acid level is increased. Because the HCO_3 level is already increased, the increased level of carbonic acid helps bring the pH level back to normal. This is

In metabolic alkalosis the respiratory system decreases its rate and depth of respirations through hypoventilation. Retaining CO_2 adds acid to the alkalotic condition.

not an efficient mechanism for reversing metabolic alkalosis because the body needs oxygen and will not obtain enough through hypoventilation. Therefore the respiratory system cannot respond in this manner for an extended period of time. The arterial blood gases of a patient with compensated metabolic alkalosis show a slightly high or normal pH level of 7.40–7.45, an increased HCO_3 (initial problem) level greater than 27 mEq/L, and an increased PCO_2 (compensatory response) greater than 45 mm Hg.

Question: Because the respiratory system responds so readily to metabolic acidosis or alkalosis, why doesn't this correct the condition?

Answer: The respiratory system is only a temporary fix for acid–base imbalances because the body fatigues. It can only hyper- or hypoventilate for a period of time before respiratory assistance is needed.

RESPIRATORY ACIDOSIS

In respiratory acidosis the kidneys work at excreting metabolic acid. The renal system is unable to eliminate carbonic acid, but the ability to eliminate other acids helps to increase the bicarbonate concentration because less is needed for buffering the excess acid. This helps to move the ratio of bicarbonate-to-carbonic acid back to 20:1. The kidneys increase the plasma bicarbonate level to greater than 27 mEq/L. The arterial blood gases of a patient with a compensated respiratory acidosis show a low or normal pH of 7.35–7.40, an elevated PCO_2 (initial problem) greater than 45 mm Hg, and an HCO_3 (compensatory mechanism) greater than 27 mEq/L.

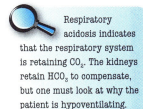

Respiratory acidosis indicates that the respiratory system is retaining CO_2. The kidneys retain HCO_3 to compensate, but one must look at why the patient is hypoventilating.

RESPIRATORY ALKALOSIS

In respiratory alkalosis the lungs excrete too much CO_2. The kidneys again attempt to compensate for the imbalance by decreasing the excretion of metabolic acid and therefore conserving acid. The renal system also attempts to decrease the bicarbonate concentration to less than 23 mEq/L. As more acid circulates in the blood in lieu of the lost carbonic acid, the bicarbonate concentration is used up with buffering. This tends to return the pH to normal. The renal system's compensatory response to respiratory alkalosis is infrequent because most of these situations are short-lived. The arterial blood gases of a patient with a compensated respiratory alkalosis show a slightly elevated or normal pH of 7.40–7.45, a PCO_2 less than 35 mm Hg, and an HCO_3 (compensatory mechanism) less than 23 mEq/L.

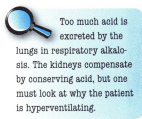

Too much acid is excreted by the lungs in respiratory alkalosis. The kidneys compensate by conserving acid, but one must look at why the patient is hyperventilating.

Mixed disturbances occur when both respiratory and metabolic disorders result in a condition of acidosis or alkalosis. How high or low the pH becomes depends on which system disturbance is most prevalent. Treatment depends on the situation and the condition. The following chapter looks at various causes of a mixed disturbance.

35

Mixed Disturbances

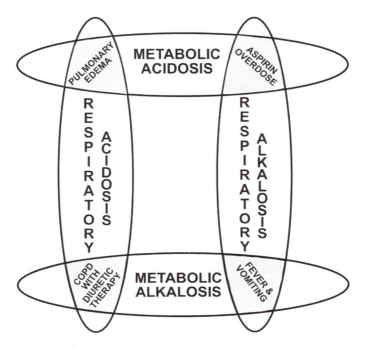

Figure 35-1 Metabolic acidosis and metabolic alkalosis.

ACID-BASE IMBALANCES

A primary acid–base imbalance occurs when an overwhelming amount of acid or base causes an imbalance with homeostasis. A metabolic acidosis occurs when the kidneys are not able to excrete enough metabolic acid or produce enough bicarbonate to equal the amount of acid. Metabolic alkalosis occurs when the kidneys produce too much bicarbonate and not enough acid is reabsorbed to counter the increased bicarbonate.

In respiratory acidosis too much carbonic acid is retained, causing a buildup of CO_2, and not enough bicarbonate exists to compensate the increased carbonic acid. Respiratory alkalosis occurs when too much carbonic acid is expelled as CO_2 and not enough metabolic acid is available to counteract for the lack of CO_2.

MIXED DISTURBANCES

A mixed acid–base disturbance is an imbalance of both the respiratory and metabolic processes. This occurs when both the respiratory and renal systems demonstrate a primary imbalance with acid or base as a response to a disease process. How high or low the pH becomes depends on which system disturbance is most prevalent. There are numerous situations in which a mixed disturbance can develop. For example, chronic obstructive pulmonary disease often manifests as a respiratory acidosis. If the patient also suffers from diabetes mellitus and currently has a severe infection or has undergone the stress of surgery, a metabolic acidosis may also occur and then a mixed disturbance exists. Both the respiratory and metabolic systems are creating an acidotic situation.

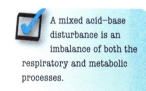

A mixed acid–base disturbance is an imbalance of both the respiratory and metabolic processes.

Another example is an elderly patient who is suffering from pneumonia, not exchanging air properly, and unable to expel secretions. The patient is given antibiotics and develops diarrhea from the medication. This patient could be in a respiratory acidosis from the pneumonia and a metabolic acidosis from the diarrhea, a mixed disturbance. Frequently, a mixed disturbance occurs with patients suffering from cardiac arrest who develop a respiratory acidosis from hypoventilation and a lactic acidosis from anaerobic metabolism.

Mixed disturbances can alter the alkaline status of the body. A patient connected to nasogastric suction loses acid along with the gastric secretions, causing metabolic alkalosis. If the patient is hyperventilating secondary to pain and losing CO_2, a respiratory alkalosis exists concurrently with the metabolic alkalosis.

Patients suffering from serious and chronic diseases suffer from mixed acid–base disorders. Mixed disturbances occur when both respiratory and metabolic disorders result in a condition of acidosis or alkalosis together. Treatment depends on the situation and the condition.

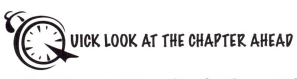

QUICK LOOK AT THE CHAPTER AHEAD

The following chapter identifies the normal laboratory values for arterial blood gases. A step-by-step process is used. Examples of acid–base imbalances are also given.

36

Arterial Blood Gas Interpretation

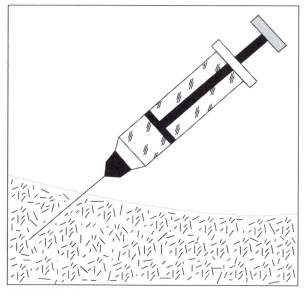

Figure 36-1 Arterial blood gas interpretation.

To interpret arterial blood gases for a patient, one must know what the normal values are:

pH   7.35–7.45
pCO_2 35–45 mm Hg
HCO_3 23–27 mEq/L

Normal arterial blood gas values are as follows:
pH   7.35–7.45
pCO_2 35–45 mm Hg
HCO_3 23–27 mEq/L

There are three steps in determining and imbalance. In the first step, always look at the pH to determine acidosis or alkalosis:

$$pH < 7.35 = acidosis$$
$$pH > 7.45 = alkalosis$$

In the second step, determine what is causing the imbalance: Is it the CO_2 or HCO_3?

$$pCO_2 < 35 \text{ mm Hg} = alkalosis$$
$$pCO_2 > 45 \text{ mm Hg} = acidosis$$

$$HCO_3 < 23 \text{ mEq/L} = acidosis$$
$$HCO_3 > 27 \text{ mEq/L} = alkalosis$$

In the third step, determine whether compensation is occurring:

    pH 7.35–7.40 = compensated acidosis

    pH 7.40–7.45 = compensated alkalosis

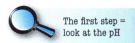

The first step =
look at the pH

The second step =
look at which system is
causing the imbalance

The third step =
is compensation occurring?

EXAMPLES OF ACID-BASE IMBALANCES

Metabolic acidosis (uncompensated):

pH = 7.32

pCO_2 = 32 mm Hg

HCO_3 = 14 mEq/L

An example of this type of imbalance is a patient suffering from chronic renal failure.

Question: The pCO_2 isn't normal. Why doesn't that result affect the equation?

Answer: Always remember to look at the pH value first. The pH of 7.32 indicates acidosis and the only value contributing to acidosis is the HCO_3. The low pCO_2 is actually a value indicating alkalosis. This arterial blood gas result could be an example of a patient suffering from chronic renal failure.

Metabolic acidosis (compensated):

pH = 7.37

pCO_2 = 28 mm Hg

HCO_3 = 21 mEq/L

Question: Why is this result considered compensated?

Answer: The pH value falls in the compensated range for metabolic acidosis. The other values can still be abnormal with a compensated pH. One of the systems (respiratory) has compensated for the out-of-normal range, the bicarbonate system. Perhaps the pCO_2 has decreased through hyperventilation to decrease the amount of H_2CO_3 in the body.

Metabolic alkalosis (uncompensated):

    pH = 7.52

    pCO_2 = 48 mm Hg

    HCO_3 = 30 mEq/L

Question: The pCO_2 is also abnormal. How does it factor into this blood gas result?

Answer: The pH indicates alkalosis, and the only result that is also indicative of alkalosis is the HCO_3. The pCO_2 is elevated because the body is attempting to hypoventilate to retain acid and compensate for the increased bicarbonate. This arterial blood gas result could be seen in a surgical patient who is losing too much acid through nasogastric suctioning.

Metabolic alkalosis (compensated):
pH = 7.44
pCO_2 = 48 mm Hg
HCO_3 = 29 mEq/L

Question: When the pH falls within the range of 7.35–7.45 is it always considered compensated even though the other values are out of range?

Answer: Yes, as long as the pH is a normal value, the body has compensated for the value that is out of range. This arterial blood gas is similar to the uncompensated metabolic alkalosis result and could be the same patient situation; however, the body has now compensated for the elevated HCO_3 by retaining acid (elevated pCO_2).

Respiratory acidosis (uncompensated):
pH = 7.33
pCO_2 = 55 mm Hg
HCO_3 = 23 mEq/L

Question: Is it truly possible for a patient to have such a high pCO_2?

Answer: Yes, frequently patients with chronic obstructive lung disease have high pCO_2 results.

Respiratory acidosis (compensated):
pH = 7.38
pCO_2 = 48 mm Hg
HCO_3 = 29 mEq/L

Question: Which system has made the pH compensated?

Answer: The metabolic system (HCO_3), has increased to compensate for the elevated respiratory system (pCO_2).

Respiratory alkalosis (uncompensated):
pH = 7.50
pCO$_2$ = 30 mm Hg
HCO$_3$ = 21 mEq/L

Question: What type of patient condition would cause respiratory alkalosis?

Answer: Any situation where the patient would hyperventilate and blow off CO$_2$, such as a patient with a hypermetabolic state such as fever or sepsis.

Respiratory alkalosis (compensated):
pH = 7.44
pCO$_2$ = 32 mm Hg
HCO$_3$ = 22 mEq/L

Question: Is this pH considered to be compensated?

Answer: Yes, it falls within the normal range of the pH values. However, the pCO$_2$ is low, indicating a respiratory alkalosis. The HCO$_3$ is slightly decreased in an attempt to decrease bicarbonate levels.

Respiratory and metabolic acidosis (mixed disturbance):
pH = 7.30
pCO$_2$ = 50 mm Hg
HCO$_3$ = 19 mEq/L

Question: What is a mixed disturbance?

Answer: A mixed disturbance occurs when both systems are out of the normal value range, resulting in an acidosis or alkalosis. An example of a patient with this type of arterial blood gas result could be one with chronic renal failure and chronic obstructive pulmonary disease.

Respiratory and metabolic alkalosis (mixed disturbance):
pH = 7.50
pCO$_2$ = 32 mm Hg
HCO$_3$ = 30 mEq/L

Question: With a mixed disturbance, do all the values need to indicate an acidosis or alkalosis?

Answer: Yes, as with this arterial blood gas result. The pCO$_2$ is low, indicating that the patient is losing acid via the respiratory system, possibly from hyperventilation or from pain, and the HCO$_3$ is elevated, indicating the patient is losing acid, perhaps from prolonged nasogastric suction (loss of HCL acid along with gastric secretions).

PART III • QUESTIONS

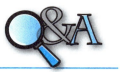

1. The more hydrogen ions in a solution the more _____ the solution.
   (A) Acidic
   (B) Base
   (C) Salty
   (D) Alkaline

2. Which of the following systems is able to eliminate carbon dioxide to maintain acid–base balance?
   (A) Renal system
   (B) Protein buffering system
   (C) Phosphate buffering system
   (D) Respiratory system

3. In a state of acidosis the _____ ion moves into the cell and the _____ ion moves out of the cell in an attempt to buffer the acidic state of the body.
   (A) Potassium, hydrogen
   (B) Sodium, chloride
   (C) Chloride, sodium
   (D) Hydrogen, potassium

4. If the pH rises, indicating an alkaline imbalance, the kidneys will
   (A) Eliminate the hydrogen ion
   (B) Attempt to hide the hydrogen ion inside the cell
   (C) Reabsorb the hydrogen ion and excrete bicarbonate
   (D) Increase production of bicarbonate

5. In a state of metabolic acidosis the patient manifests which of the following respiration patterns?
   (A) Deep and rapid
   (B) Slow and shallow
   (C) Cluster
   (D) Cheyne-Stokes

6. The compensatory mechanism for metabolic alkalosis is
   (A) Hyperventilation
   (B) Renal excretion of acid
   (C) Hypoventilation
   (D) Renal production and reabsorption of bicarbonate

7. A patient with chronic lung disease becomes conditioned to an elevated _____ level in the blood.
   (A) Oxygen
   (B) Carbon dioxide
   (C) Hydrogen
   (D) Potassium

8. What condition occurs when too much carbonic acid is expelled during expiration?
   (A) Respiratory acidosis
   (B) Metabolic acidosis
   (C) Metabolic alkalosis
   (D) Respiratory alkalosis

9. The following arterial blood gas results of pH = 7.32, pCO_2 = 49 mm Hg, and HCO_3 mEq/L = 25 indicate
   (A) Respiratory alkalosis
   (B) Metabolic alkalosis
   (C) Respiratory acidosis
   (D) Metabolic acidosis

10. Which of the following arterial blood gas results indicates a mixed disturbance?
   (A) pH = 7.50, pCO_2 = 32 mm Hg, HCO_3 = 32 mEq/L
   (B) pH = 7.30, pCO_2 = 50 mm Hg, HCO_3 = 29 mEq/L
   (C) pH = 7.45, pCO_2 = 45 mm Hg, HCO_3 = 23 mEq/L
   (D) pH = 7.52, pCO_2 = 47 mm Hg, HCO_3 = 29 mEq/L

PART III • ANSWERS AND RATIONALES

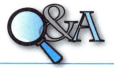

1. The correct answer is A.
   Rationale: Hydrogen is an acid; therefore, the more hydrogen ions in a solution the more acidic the solution, and the less hydrogen ions in a solution the more alkaline the solution.

2. The correct answer is D.
   Rationale: Only the respiratory system can expel acid through respiration in an attempt to correct an acid imbalance. The protein and phosphate systems will attempt to buffer excess acid in the body. The renal system will produce bicarbonate as a buffering mechanism.

3. The correct answer is D.
   Rationale: The hydrogen ion (acid) will move into the cell in exchange for the potassium ion. This is an attempt to hide the acid inside the cell as the body attempts to buffer or eliminate the remaining acid.

4. The correct answer is C.
   Rationale: In an alkaline state, the kidneys will attempt to retain acid (hydrogen ion) and eliminate bicarbonate. Eliminating the hydrogen ion or hiding it inside the cell only increases the alkaline state. Increasing production of bicarbonate also adds base and increases the state of alkalinity.

5. The correct answer is A.
   Rationale: In a state of metabolic acidosis, the individual will attempt to rid the body of excess acid (carbon dioxide) through deep and rapid (Kussmaul) respirations. Slow and shallow breathing only increases the amount of carbon dioxide. Cluster breathing is an irregular pattern of cluster breaths with occasional periods of apnea. A Cheyne-Stokes pattern of breathing is a pattern of crescendo–decrescendo respirations accompanied by periods of apnea.

6. The correct answer is C.
   Rationale: The retention of carbon dioxide (acid) through hypoventilation helps to increase the acid content of the blood. Hyperventilation only increases the alkaline state by eliminating carbon dioxide. Eliminating the hydrogen ion (acid) through the renal system or retaining bicarbonate (base) also only increases the alkalinity.

7. The correct answer is B.
   Rationale: Alveolar ventilation is impaired in the patient with chronic lung disease. This causes an increase in carbon dioxide. The medullary system becomes accustomed to the elevated pCO_2 levels and the patient's respiratory drive can actually become suppressed from elevated O_2 administration.

8. The correct answer is D.
   Rationale: Respiratory alkalosis occurs when too much carbon dioxide is expelled, such as with conditions of hyperventilation. The renal system cannot expel carbon dioxide, and respiratory acidosis is an accumulation of too much carbon dioxide.

9. The correct answer is C.
   Rationale: The pH indicates a state of acidosis, the CO_2 is elevated, indicating increased carbon dioxide in the blood, and the bicarbonate level is normal.

10. The correct answer is A.
    Rationale: Both the respiratory and metabolic systems reflect a state of alkalosis. Answer B is a respiratory acidosis. Answer C is normal. Answer D is only a metabolic alkalosis.

IV

Organ Systems Control

QUICK LOOK AT THE CHAPTER AHEAD

The hypothalamus is the most important organ responsible for maintaining homeostasis. In this chapter we briefly explain the functions of the thirst center and the antidiuretic hormone.

37

Hypothalamus and Fluid Regulation

Hypothalamus

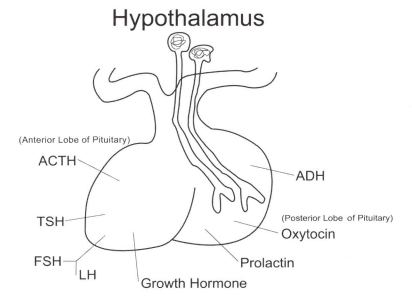

(Anterior Lobe of Pituitary)
ACTH

ADH

TSH

(Posterior Lobe of Pituitary)
Oxytocin

FSH
LH
Growth Hormone

Prolactin

Figure 37-1 The hypothalamus.

The hypothalamus is the most important organ responsible for maintaining homeostasis (Figure 37-1). Its control over the respiratory and cardiovascular systems and stress, metabolic, and fluid and electrolyte balance is essential for supporting life. The hypothalamus is connected to and controls the pituitary gland, which has two lobes, the anterior lobe (adenohypophysis) and the posterior lobe (neurohypophysis). The anterior lobe is known as the master gland and conducts multiple functions through specialized cells that secrete specific hormones for particular metabolic roles. The posterior lobe, however, communicates with the hypothalamus in the regulation of fluid balance with **antidiuretic hormone (ADH)**, or vasopressin. The hypothalamus synthesizes ADH, which is transported and stored in the neurohypophysis until its needed release for fluid regulation. A system of feedback loops is used to regulate the posterior pituitary gland to release ADH, which affects the target organ, producing the desired physiological response.

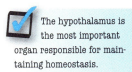

The hypothalamus is the most important organ responsible for maintaining homeostasis.

THIRST

Extremely sensitive **osmoreceptors** located near or in the thirst center of the hypothalamus are responsible for sensing the need for water. They have the capability to respond to changes in the osmolality of the extracellular compartment. When an increase in osmolality occurs the cells dehydrate, which triggers the osmoreceptors to prompt the individual to take in water until the thirst center is satisfied. It is possible that the thirst center is connected to the storage and release area for ADH, accounting for the close relationship between the two.

 When an increase in osmolality occurs the cells dehydrate, which triggers the osmoreceptors to prompt the individual to take in water until the thirst center is satisfied.

ANTIDIURETIC HORMONE

The primary function of ADH is to regulate fluid volume based on the amount that can be absorbed via the renal tubules. Whether the initiator is decreased extracellular fluid or an increased sodium concentration, ADH helps to replenish the fluid loss and to regain homeostatic balance.

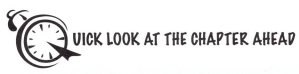

The function of the kidneys is to remove and add substances to and from the blood through glomerular filtration, tubular reabsorption, and tubular secretion. These three functions are described here, along with fluid regulation, conservation, and elimination.

38

Kidney Regulation of Electrolytes and Fluid

TERMS
- ☐ **Atrial natriuretic peptide (ANP)**
- ☐ **Glomerular filtration**

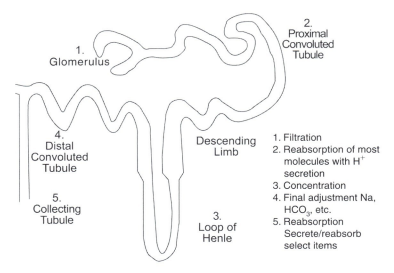

Figure 38-1 Kidney regulation.

Kidneys remove and add substances to and from the blood through glomerular filtration, tubular reabsorption, and tubular secretion. Their ability to reabsorb and secrete electrolytes, maintain an acid–base balance, and conserve or eliminate water is a remarkable system of checks and balances.

GLOMERULAR FILTRATION

Glomerular filtration involves the filtering of fluids and solutes. Protein and blood cells are too large to pass through the glomerular filtration membrane barrier; therefore the filtrate is a protein-free fluid with the same composition as plasma. In the healthy individual this filtrate is isoosmotic at approximately 300 mOsm/L. Approximately 180 L of glomerulate filtrate is formed each day. Of this filtrate, 99% is reabsorbed and 1 to 2 L is considered urine output each day.

TUBULAR REABSORPTION

The kidneys have the ability to change the acid–base balance or composition of electrolytes in the plasma by changing the composition of the glomerular filtrate through **tubular reabsorption**. Active and passive transport are the mechanisms of movement of molecules in the tubules. Some electrolytes passively ride on sodium (cotransport) as it is actively transported through the system. Other ions transport themselves through osmosis or diffusion in passive transport. As solutes become more concentrated on one side of the tubules and the other side becomes less concentrated, fluid flows to the area of increased concentration. This helps to maintain a normal plasma osmolarity.

Question: How does tubular reabsorption occur?

Answer: Tubular reabsorption occurs through both active and passive transport.

TUBULAR SECRETION

Substances move from the peritubular capillaries into the lumen of the tubule through active secretion. Both organic acids and bases are transported in this manner. Various molecules, drugs, toxins, and metabolic wastes can be excreted via the pumping action of **tubular secretion**.

CONCENTRATION OF GLOMERULAR FILTRATE AS IT TRAVELS THROUGH THE NEPHRON

Urine formation starts as the filtrate is formed in the glomerulus. This filtrate is a protein-free plasma that travels through the tubules and ducts of the nephron. Approximately 65% of reabsorption and secretion of electrolytes, vitamins, and amino acids takes place in the proximal tubules of the kidney. Sodium and potassium are actively transported from the proximal collecting tubule into the capillaries. The movement of the two cations allows for negative ions such as Cl^- and HPO_4^{2-} to passively flow along to maintain electroneutrality. Hydrogen is actively exchanged for Na^+ in the proximal tubule and then is allowed to combine with HCO_3^- to form H_2CO_3. Carbonic acid readily breaks down into H_2O and CO_2, which diffuse and, along with the enzyme carbonic anhydrase, again form HCO_3^- and H^+ (Figure 38-2). The bicarbonate combines with Na^+ and the H^+ is secreted to be again reabsorbed as H_2O.

$$CO_2 + H_2O \leftrightarrow H_2CO_3 \leftrightarrow H^+ + HCO_3^-$$

Figure 38-2 Carbonic acid–bicarbonate buffering system.

The isoosmotic glomerular filtrate passes from the proximal collecting tubule to the descending limb of the loop of Henle. As it moves down the loop it meets with highly osmotic fluid in the medulla. The descending limb, under the influence of the antidiuretic hormone (ADH), is readily permeable to water; therefore the highly osmotic fluid initiates an osmotic movement of water out of the filtrate and the passive diffusion of Na^+ and Cl^- into the filtrate. The filtrate is hyperosmolar at approximately 1,200 mOsm/L as it begins to turn up the ascending limb of the loop of Henle. Unlike the descending limb, however, the ascending limb is impermeable to water. Solutes such as Na^+, Cl^-, and K^+ are readily reabsorbed here, but water cannot follow the ions. This makes the filtrate more dilute to the point of being hypoosmolar. Traveling to the distal convoluted tubule, water continues to meet the barrier of impermeable tubules. Sodium and chloride reabsorption continues, contributing to the decreased osmolarity of the already dilute filtrate.

As the filtrate travels to the late distal and cortical collecting tubules, aldosterone, a hormone secreted by the adrenal gland (see Chapter 8), exerts its effect on sodium reabsorption. This area is also a primary site for potassium excretion. Although potassium and sodium are excreted and reabsorbed along the journey through the glomerulus and nephron, the distal and cortical collecting tubules become the final place where the concentration of these two important electrolytes for the body is determined.

FLUID REGULATION

During periods of dehydration or fluid excess, the kidneys work hard to maintain fluid balance. Whichever situation exists, the medullary collecting duct is where the fluid becomes highly concentrated or diluted. This is also where it becomes highly acidic or alkaline.

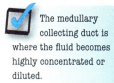

The medullary collecting duct is where the fluid becomes highly concentrated or diluted.

Fluid Conservation

ADH influences the regulation of fluid at the medullary collecting duct. If a need for fluid is sensed by the osmoreceptors, ADH is released by the neurohypophysis (posterior pituitary), sodium is reabsorbed, and the kidneys retain fluid.

Another influence on fluid balance is the renin-angiotensin-aldosterone system. When blood flow decreases, renin, an enzyme stored in the kidneys, is released. Through an enzyme-converting mechanism, it acts on angiotensinogen to become angiotensin I. Angiotensin I circulates to the lungs and meets with an angiotensin-converting enzyme to become angiotensin II. Angiotensin II has the property of stimulating aldosterone to increase sodium reabsorption. In addition, angiotensin II has the ability to vasoconstrict the efferent arteriole, allowing for an increased glomerular filtration pressure and maintenance of fluid volume.

Fluid Elimination

Atrial natriuretic peptide (ANP) is another hormone that affects salt and water balance. Synthesized in the atrium of the heart, it is released when the muscle cells of the heart become stretched from too much volume. ANP aids in decreasing the amount of blood return to the heart through vasodilation of the blood vessels, which in turn affects the efferent and afferent arterioles of the kidney. This helps to increase the glomerular filtration rate. In addition, ANP inhibits the release of aldosterone and ADH, which prevents the reabsorption of sodium and water.

In this chapter we examine the passage of carbon dioxide through the respiratory system, the movement of chloride as it shifts into the cell for electrical neutrality, and the role of the respiratory system in balancing fluids.

39

Respiratory Regulation of Carbon Dioxide and Fluids

TERMS
☐ **Chloride shift**

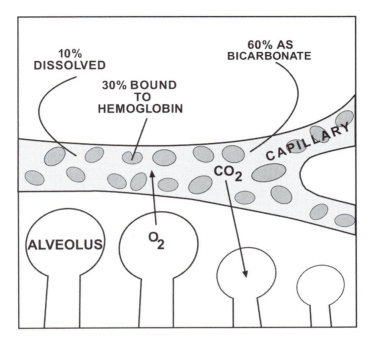

Figure 39-1 Respiratory regulation of carbon dioxide and fluids.

CARBON DIOXIDE

Through the process of breathing, a combination of oxygen and nitrogen gases enters the respiratory system. As the gases travel the vascular system, carbon dioxide travels the opposite pathway in exchange for oxygen. Carbon dioxide diffuses into the capillary at the venous end and returns to the lungs via the pulmonary artery and arterioles. Once in the pulmonary bed, it diffuses across the alveolar–capillary interspace to enter the alveolus for expiration. Approximately 10% of carbon dioxide travels in its dissolved state in plasma. It is the dissolved CO_2 that is measured as the pCO_2 with a range of 35–45 mm Hg. This range closely resembles that of the partial pressure of gases in the alveoli. Any increase in the amount of CO_2 easily can tilt the pH balance to an acidic state. Just as easily, any decrease in CO_2 can result in an increase in alkalinity. Of the remaining carbon dioxide, 30% is attached to hemoglobin and 60% is transported as bicarbonate. The dissolved CO_2 is carried to the alveoli of the lungs while the remaining diffuses into tissue spaces and capillaries.

Chloride Shift

Carbon dioxide prefers to combine with hemoglobin in the red blood cell or with carbonic acid. As mentioned previously, the $H_2CO_3^-$ easily ionizes to HCO_3^- and H^+. The hydrogen ion is allowed to combine with hemoglobin, Hb^-, to form hydrogen hemoglobin, HHb, a buffer for acid–base alterations. If large amounts of bicarbonate are drawn into the plasma and a negative charge is needed in the red blood cell for equalization, Cl^- moves into the cell. This movement, referred to as a **chloride shift**, allows for increased amount of bicarbonate to move into the plasma to act as a buffering mechanism while chloride maintains electrical neutrality within the cell.

Within the respiratory system, attempts to rectify acid–base imbalances occur rapidly. The hydrogen hemoglobin molecule splits to release H^+ so it can bond with bicarbonate again and form carbonic acid. This combination rapidly breaks into water and CO_2, which can be expelled during expiration to help decrease acid or kept to increase the acid balance. Chemoreceptors, sensitive to carbon dioxide changes, are located in the medulla of the brain. They respond to an increased metabolic state by causing an increased formation of carbon dioxide. In addition, if metabolism decreases, carbon dioxide formation decreases. In this manner, the respiratory rate increases or decreases depending on the underlying cause.

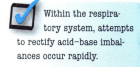 Within the respiratory system, attempts to rectify acid–base imbalances occur rapidly.

RESPIRATORY FLUID LOSS

During expiration, water is expelled along with gases. If hyperventilation exists for a significant period of time, even though the fluid loss is not in large amounts, this loss can contribute to an already compromised fluid balance. In addition, the mouth, nose, and airway passages also become dried, making defense against debris removal and antimicrobial agents difficult.

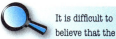 It is difficult to believe that the respiratory system has much to do with fluid balance, but for the already compromised patient hyperventilation can easily contribute to a state of dehydration due to water being expelled along with respiratory gases.

Humidified oxygen delivery is of high importance to prevent drying of the respiratory system.

Fluid loss can also occur via the respiratory system by leakage out of the pulmonary capillaries. This is normally prevented through osmotic pressures and capillary hydrostatic pressure. However, fluid overload may cause fluid to leak into the alveoli and tissue interstitium, causing decreased diffusion of gases essential for breathing. This is discussed further in Part V, Chapters 44 and 45.

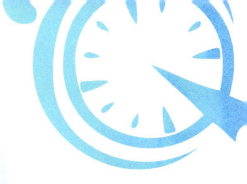

Part of the integumentary system, the skin is the largest organ in the body, protecting the musculoskeletal structure and internal organs. In this chapter we discuss the qualities of skin and how fluid is lost through the skin.

40

Skin as a Barrier to Fluid Loss

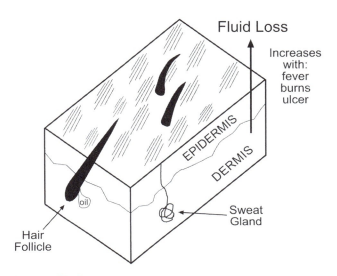

Figure 40-1 Skin as a barrier to fluid loss.

The skin is the largest organ in the body, protecting the musculoskeletal structure and internal organs. The skin, hair, nails, glands, and nerves, known as the integumentary system, make up an intricate structure that helps to regulate body temperature, fluid loss, production of vitamin D, and microbial defense. It comprises 20% of the body's weight. The skin has an elastic quality that allows for stretching. It is thick and tough in some areas, such as the palms of the hands and soles of the feet, and smooth and silky in others, such as the mucous membranes of the mouth and eyelids.

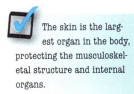 The skin is the largest organ in the body, protecting the musculoskeletal structure and internal organs.

FLUID LOSS THROUGH THE SKIN

Along with its many other functions the skin is waterproof, yet it allows for perspiration to help regulate body temperature. Through its peripheral thermoreceptors, the skin has an ability to trigger the hypothalamus for heat production and conservation when the temperature is low and evaporation when the temperature is hot. An increase in perspiration through the skin surface and mucous membrane linings aids in body water evaporation. Excessive perspiration, however, can affect the body's fluid balance and electrolyte status.

Burns can cause a rapid fluid loss through the skin. Fluid seeps out of open skin and also seeps into the tissues. The amount of protein loss affects the loss of fluid. With the loss of protein, altered colloid osmotic pressure, and increased capillary permeability, fluid shifts, causing edema.

Question: **How do burns cause a fluid shift in the body?**

Answer: **When protein is lost through leaky capillaries, the colloidal osmotic pressure is no longer able to pull fluid back into the capillary, resulting in a loss of fluid.**

Pressure ulcers and fistulas also affect water loss. Pressure sores form in vulnerable patients with compromised peripheral circulation or the inability to move and change positions normally. Compressing the skin so that the capillary pressure exceeds 25 mm Hg occludes blood vessels in the tissue. Frequent repositioning helps to relieve this pressure, but when repositioning is not performed ulcers begin to form. Constant weeping from large pressure ulcers and fistulas can affect the body's fluid balance.

Trauma such as deep puncture wounds, facial lacerations, and open compound fractures cause an opening in the skin for blood loss. Major trauma can affect the body's fluid balance until replacement fluid has been administered and the skin repaired.

Excessive perspiration, burns, pressure ulcers, fistulas, and major trauma can cause fluid loss through the skin, contributing to a compromised fluid balance.

PART IV · QUESTIONS

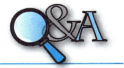

1. One of the major hormones released by the hypothalamus/
   pituitary is
   (A) Renin
   (B) ADH
   (C) ANP
   (D) Creatine

2. The descending limb of the loop of Henle is readily_____ to
   water and the ascending limb of the loop of Henle is _____to
   water.
   (A) Permeable/impermeable
   (B) Impermeable/permeable

3. Which of the following systems is the quickest responder to an
   acid–base imbalance?
   (A) Renal system
   (B) Protein buffering system
   (C) Phosphate buffering system
   (D) Respiratory system

4. Which of the following is *not* a source of fluid loss through the
   skin?
   (A) Deep puncture wounds
   (B) Open compound fractures
   (C) Exhalation
   (D) Burns

5. Which of the following is the *best* communicator with the hypo-
   thalamus in the regulation of fluid balance?
   (A) Posterior lobe of the pituitary gland
   (B) Renal system
   (C) Dehydrated cells
   (D) Increased osmolality

6. Glomerular filtration involves the filtering of _____ and _____.
   (A) Protein, blood cells
   (B) Blood cells, electrolytes
   (C) Electrolytes, protein
   (D) Fluids, solutes

7. When is ANP released for water balance?
   (A) For fluid conservation
   (B) With increased osmolality
   (C) When the muscle cells of the heart become stretched from too much volume
   (D) After the release of renin

8. An increase in CO_2 beyond 45 mm Hg will _____ the pH balance to an _____ state.
   (A) Increase, alkalotic
   (B) Decrease, alkalotic
   (C) Decrease, acidotic
   (D) Increase, acidotic

9. The largest organ in the body is the
   (A) Liver
   (B) Heart
   (C) Brain
   (D) Skin

10. Osmoreceptors located near or in the thirst center are responsible for sensing the need for _____.
   (A) O_2
   (B) Water
   (C) CO_2
   (D) An increase in temperature

PART IV · ANSWERS AND RATIONALES

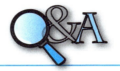

1. The correct answer is B.
   Rationale: ADH is released by the hypothalamus/posterior pituitary in response to an increased osmolality. Renin is initiated by the renal system in response to a need for vasoconstriction. ANP is synthesized in the atrium of the heart in response to an increased fluid volume. Creatine is a byproduct of muscle catabolism.

2. The correct answer is A.
   Rationale: The descending limb is readily permeable to water, which helps with the passive diffusion of sodium and chloride into the filtrate. The ascending limb is impermeable to water, which keeps the filtrate in a hypoosmolar state.

3. The correct answer is B.
   Rationale: Proteins are the largest system for buffering, acting as either an acid or a base, and are immediately available to combine to either excess acid or base imbalances in the body. The respiratory system is a fast responder to an acid–base imbalance through its ability to expel carbon dioxide. The renal system is the slowest, taking days to weeks. The phosphate buffering system works best when the renal tubular fluid is flooded with excess H^+ ions.

4. The correct answer is C.
   Rationale: Trauma such as deep puncture wounds, open compound fractures, and burns involve openings in the skin where fluid can escape. Fluid is lost through exhalation, but exhalation is a function of the respiratory system, not the integumentary.

5. The correct answer is A.
   Rationale: The posterior lobe of the pituitary communicates directly with the hypothalamus with the hormone ADH or vasopressin in the regulation of fluid balance. The renal system works hard to maintain fluid balance through conserving or eliminating fluid. Dehydrated cells and an increased osmolality are symptoms that trigger the hypothalamus to begin fluid regulation.

6. The correct answer is D.
   Rationale: Glomerular filtration involves the filtering of fluids and solutes. Protein and blood cells are too large to pass through the glomerular filtration membrane, making the filtrate protein free.

7. The correct answer is C.
   Rationale: ANP is a hormone that affects water balance and is released when the heart muscle cells are overstretched from too much volume. It helps to vasodilate the blood vessels, which helps increase the glomerular filtration rate. A decreased fluid balance or increased osmolality indicate low fluid volume. The release of renin begins a cycle of vasoconstriction to maintain fluid volume.

8. The correct answer is C.
   Rationale: An increase in the CO_2, which is an acid, decreases the pH value and contributes to an acidotic state.

9. The correct answer is D.
   Rationale: The skin is the largest organ in the body, protecting the musculoskeletal structure and internal organs, and has multiple functions.

10. The correct answer is B.
    Rationale: The osmoreceptors located near or in the thirst center of the hypothalamus are responsible for sensing the need for water. They respond to an increase in osmolality. They are not responsible for gases or temperature.

V

Fluid and Electrolyte Balance in Disease Processes and Nursing Implications

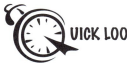

QUICK LOOK AT THE CHAPTER AHEAD

Acute renal failure is related to a sudden decrease in the glomerular filtration rate, causing a low urine output. Prerenal, intrarenal, or postrenal factors as causes for acute renal failure are examined here. The three stages of acute renal failure are also discussed, along with treatment and nursing implications.

41
Acute Renal Failure

TERMS
☐ **Acute renal failure**

CAUSES	MANIFESTATIONS
PRERENAL	**STAGE 1**
HYPOVOLEMIA SHOCK ARTERIAL/ VENOUS OBSTRUCTION	90% OLIGURIC LOSE SODIUM GRADIENT BUN/CR RISE 1-7 DAYS
INTRARENAL	**STAGE 2**
GLOMERULONEPHRITIS NEPHROTOXIC AGENTS HEMOGLOBINURIA MYOGLOBINURIA IMMUNE/INFILTRATIVE	EARLY DIURESIS LARGE SHIFTS OF FLUIDS SEEN 1-3 WEEKS
POSTRENAL	**STAGE 3**
TUMOR OBSTRUCTION ENLARGED PROSTATE CALCULI TRAUMA	3-12 MONTHS 30% WITHOUT RECOVERY

Figure 41-1 Causes and manifestations of acute renal failure.

CAUSES OF ACUTE RENAL FAILURE

Acute renal failure is related to a sudden decrease in the glomerular filtration rate, causing a low urine output. It is treatable and reversible. The etiology of renal failure may be due to prerenal, intrarenal, or postrenal factors.

Prerenal Factors

Prerenal causes of acute renal failure occur as situations outside of the renal system that decrease pressure in the afferent arteriole and consequently restrict blood flow to the kidneys. Though compensatory measures help to maintain blood flow to the kidneys, an arterial pressure of less than 70 mm Hg causes most compensatory mechanisms to

 Prerenal causes of acute renal failure occur as situations outside of the renal system that decrease pressure in the afferent arteriole and consequently restrict blood flow to the kidneys.

fail. Cardiovascular disorders, low blood volume, drugs causing vasoconstriction or peripheral dilation, or obstruction to the renal vasculature such as clamping major arteries during surgery are some of the factors related to decreasing the blood flow to the kidneys. If blood flow is restored in time, damage caused by these situations is minimal.

Intrarenal Factors

Intrarenal factors cause damage to the renal tissue and nephrons of the kidneys. The glomerulus may be the site of injury, such as with glomerulonephritis, but most commonly acute tubular necrosis is the cause of acute

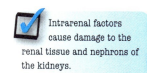

Intrarenal factors cause damage to the renal tissue and nephrons of the kidneys.

renal failure. Acute tubular necrosis can be caused by either prerenal or postrenal factors if they result in ischemia or nephrotoxic damage to the tubules. Nephrotoxic injury may be caused by aminoglycoside antibiotics or radiocontrast dyes. Hemoglobin released from damaged red blood cells (caused by mismatched blood transfusions) or myoglobin released from crushed muscle cells (rhabdomyolysis) combined in a series of events has a direct toxic effect, causing damage to the tubular cell.

Question: What is the most common cause of acute renal failure?

Answer: Acute tubular necrosis.

Postrenal Factors

Postrenal factors responsible for acute renal failure include damage that occurs to the structures located distal to the kidneys. An obstruction to urine flow, whether located in the bladder, ureters, or urethra, can result

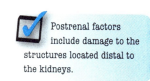

Postrenal factors include damage to the structures located distal to the kidneys.

in a backflow of urine to the kidneys, causing an increase in interstitial pressure and ultimately in the nephron. Prostatic hyperplasia, calculi, tumors, or trauma are some of the problems that can cause an obstruction to these urological structures.

CLINICAL MANIFESTATIONS OF ACUTE RENAL FAILURE

There are several stages in acute renal failure. The first stage is oliguria, which occurs in 1 to 7 days, depending on the initial insult. The second stage is diuresis, and the third stage is recovery.

Stage One: Oliguria

Oliguria Secondary to Prerenal Causes
Oliguria is the first stage of acute renal failure. Prerenal failure results from episodes related to decreased kidney perfusion (decreased pressure in the afferent arteriole) secondary to a decreased circulating blood volume to the kidney. Consequently, the body compensates through vasoconstriction and sodium and water retention. Therefore oliguria secondary to prerenal causes in acute renal failure is demonstrated by urine with a high specific gravity, high osmolality, and low sodium content. There is little damage to the infrastructure of the kidney, and the autoregulatory mechanisms of the kidneys are able to compensate (Table 41-1).

Oliguria Secondary to Intrarenal Causes
In contrast, the urine in oliguria related to intrarenal causes has a decreased specific gravity, decreased osmolality, the presence of casts, and an increased sodium. These results are related to the damaged tubules that cannot respond to correction and concentrate the urine.

Serum sodium cannot be conserved for long due to the damaged tubules and eventually levels fall. Care must be taken in evaluating the sodium levels, however, because they may actually be elevated but reflect a low value due to the increase in fluid (dilutional hypernatremia). Because

Table 41-1 Oliguria in Acute Renal Failure

Prerenal Causes	Intrarenal Causes
↑ Specific gravity	↓ Specific gravity
↑ Osmolality	↓ Osmolality
↓ Sodium content	↑ Sodium content
Little damage to kidney infrastructure	Damage to tubules
Autoregulatory mechanisms intact	Autoregulatory mechanisms *not* intact

↑ Increased; ↓ decreased.

retention of fluid volume in excess is occurring at the same time, sodium should not be replaced. Volume excess may manifest as a bounding pulse, distended neck veins, or hypertension. If allowed to progress, congestive heart failure or pulmonary edema may develop.

Question: What will my patient exhibit if he or she has fluid volume excess?

Answer: Patients with excessive fluid may have distended neck veins, an elevated blood pressure, or a bounding pulse. Those with poor hearts may develop pulmonary edema.

Because of the damaged tubules, ammonia cannot be synthesized for H^+ excretion. Consequently, acidosis occurs due to accumulation of the H^+. The respiratory system will attempt to compensate through rapid and deep (Kussmaul) respirations in an effort to blow off carbon dioxide. Bicarbonate is available for buffering the H^+, but supplies eventually diminish because the kidneys cannot replenish the quantity needed due to structural damage.

Several conditions exist to elevate the potassium level in acute renal failure. Potassium is normally lost through the urine. When output is impaired, potassium levels increase. In addition, if the acute failure is due to tissue injury, potassium is released from the damaged cells, contributing to the elevated level. The exchange of intracellular potassium for H^+ in acidosis also assists in elevating the potassium level (see Chapter 27).

The kidneys are responsible for activating vitamin D. Vitamin D is necessary for absorption of calcium from the gastrointestinal tract. If the kidneys are not functioning properly, they cannot activate vitamin D, allowing for the development of hypocalcemia.

The blood urea nitrogen and creatinine levels also elevate, resulting in azotemia. These laboratory values are reflective of urea and nitrogenous wastes, which the kidneys normally excrete. Again, because the kidneys are not working to clear the wastes, the end products of metabolism accumulate.

Stage Two: Diuresis

Because of the increased urea concentration, an osmotic diuresis occurs and eventually the urine output increases. In addition, the nephrons have not regained normal functioning capacity and cannot concentrate the urine. These two factors combined contribute to a high urine output that increases excessively to as much as 3–5 L/day. The loss of this amount of fluid may produce hypovolemia and dehydration. Electrolytes are now being lost through the high urine output; therefore hypokalemia and hyponatremia may result. The patient may manifest signs of cardiac irritability and/or hypotension. The diuretic phase may last from 1 to 3 weeks before recovery begins to occur.

Care must be taken to prevent the patient from becoming dehydrated secondary to hypovolemia when the diuretic phase of acute renal failure occurs.

Stage Three: Recovery

As the diuresis stage ends electrolyte, acid–base, and fluid balances begin to return to normal. It may take up to a year for the kidneys to regain complete function. Much depends on the overall health of the patient. If the patient is elderly and age has contributed to decreased renal perfusion and function, normal kidney function may never be regained.

Question: How does acute renal failure progress?

Answer: It progresses through three different stages. In the first stage the patient experiences oliguria, the second stage is manifested by diuresis, and finally in the third stage the patient hopefully recovers normal renal function.

TREATMENT AND NURSING IMPLICATIONS

Monitoring the patient's fluid and electrolyte status during the oliguric and diuretic phases of acute renal failure is of primary importance. Accurate measurement of intake and output, along with daily weights, should be recorded. One should be alert for the signs and symptoms of hypervolemia and hypovolemia as the condition progresses through the various stages. Laboratory values and signs and symptoms of hypernatremia versus hyponatremia, hyperkalemia versus hypokalemia, hypocalcemia, and azotemia should be assessed. Acid–base balance must be monitored to avoid the progression of acidosis and the domino effect of electrolyte imbalance that follows. Prevention of infection through asepsis of invasive lines, tubes, and procedures is of paramount importance. Infection can be life threatening because of the compromised condition of the patient. Teaching the patient to comply with the treatment regimen, especially with an antibiotic regimen, is important for complete recovery.

 Infection can be life threatening because of the compromised condition of the patient.

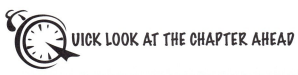

Chronic renal failure results when there is irreversible destruction of the nephrons of both kidneys and a glomerular filtration rate < 15 mL/min. In this chapter we take an in-depth look at the clinical manifestations of fluid imbalance, metabolic acidosis, and the electrolyte disturbances that occur with chronic renal failure. Treatment and nursing implications are also discussed.

42

Chronic Renal Failure

TERMS
☐ **Chronic renal failure**

CAUSES | MANIFESTATIONS

VASCULAR | FLUID BALANCE

ARTERIAL BLOCKAGE
VENOUS OCCLUSION
DIABETIC GLOMERULOSCLEROSIS
post ATN

VARIABLE OUTPUT
HYPERVOLEMIA
PERIPHERAL EDEMA

INTRARENAL

GLOMERULONEPHRITIS
TOXINS / MEDICATIONS
IMMUNE
   (GOODPASTURE'S)
RENAL CELL CARCINOMA
NEPHROSIS

METABOLIC

ACIDOSIS THAT IS ONLY
SLOWLY COMPENSATED

ELECTROLYTES

POSTRENAL

TUMOR OBSTRUCTION
CALCULI

HYPERKALEMIA
HIGH PHOSPHATE
LOW CALCIUM
HIGH MAGNESIUM
DILUTIONAL LOW Na

Figure 42-1 Causes and manifestations of chronic renal failure.

CAUSES OF CHRONIC RENAL FAILURE

In **chronic renal failure** the glomeruli slowly sclerose, the tubules atrophy, and an interstitial fibrosis occurs. The nephrons eventually become damaged and can no longer function because they are replaced by scar tissue. The glomerular filtration rate falls to < 15 mL/min. Surprisingly, however, it takes up to 80% of nephron damage before renal function becomes clinically evident. The slow progress of this process may be caused by chronic obstruction from calculi, glomerulonephritis, or pyelonephritis. Long-term use of aminoglycoside antibiotics can result in nephrotoxicity. Diabetic nephropathy can cause chronic renal failure as well as hypertension and other vascular diseases.

Question: What is the difference between acute and chronic renal failure?

Answer: Acute renal failure occurs secondary to an acute event and renal function returns to normal after the oliguric, diuretic, and recovery stages. Chronic renal failure occurs over time as the nephrons become permanently damaged. The kidneys do not return to normal function with chronic renal failure.

CLINICAL MANIFESTATIONS OF CHRONIC RENAL FAILURE

End-stage renal failure is a multisystem disease. Multiple metabolic disturbances contribute to clinical manifestations with every system of the body (Table 42-1). There is no cure for renal failure other than kidney transplant provided the patient is a candidate for that procedure. Before that stage dialysis helps to keep the patient alive.

Fluid Imbalance

Unlike acute renal failure, classified by stages, chronic renal failure is progressive, beginning with a diminished renal reserve that progresses to renal insufficiency and ultimately results in end-stage renal disease. Even with a diminished renal reserve, the kidneys maintain a sufficient glomerular filtration rate to keep the serum creatinine and blood urea nitrogen levels normal. As the ability of the kidneys to concentrate urine diminishes urine output increases; this is one of the initial signs of the beginning of the disease process. Dehydration occurs if the condition goes unattended.

The progression of the disease eventually leads to a decreased number of functioning nephrons. Interestingly, the nephron is such a viable unit that dialysis is not required until almost 90% are lost. This is due to the ability of the remaining nephrons to hypertrophy and compensate for the decrease in nephron numbers. As the disease progresses the urine is no longer dilute, urine output decreases, and, if intake exceeds output, hypervolemia occurs. The ability to clear urea and other metabolic products diminishes. The progression to end-stage renal failure is reflected as a creatinine clearance of 10 mL/min compared with a normal clearance of 85 to 135 mL/min.

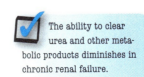
The ability to clear urea and other metabolic products diminishes in chronic renal failure.

Table 42-1 Metabolic Disturbances of Chronic Renal Failure

Psychological	**Cardiovascular**
Denial	Hypertension
Anxiety	Congestive heart failure
Depression	Pericardial effusion
Psychosis	Myocardiopathy
	Pericarditis
	Atherosclerotic heart disease, hyperlipidemia
Neurological	**Ocular**
Fatigue	Hypertensive retinopathy
Headache	
Sleep disturbances	
Lethargy	
Muscular irritability	
Seizures	
Confusion	
Coma	
Pulmonary	**Gastrointestinal**
Pulmonary edema	Anorexia
Dyspnea	Nausea/vomiting
Pneumonia	Gastritis/stomatitis
Uremic lung	Peptic ulcer
	GI bleed
	Metallic taste in mouth
	Nutritional deficiencies
Endocrine	**Reproductive**
Hyperparathyroidism	Infertility
Thyroid dysfunction	Sexual dysfunction
	Azoospermia
	Amenorrhea
Integumentary	**Metabolic**
Pruritus/dry skin	Gout
Pallor/pigmentation changes	
Ecchymosis/excoriations	
Uremic frost	
Peripheral Neuropathy	**Hematological**
Paresthesias	Anemia
Motor weakness	Bleeding
Restless leg syndrome	Infection

Metabolic Acidosis

The kidneys normally excrete a significant amount of acid on a daily basis. An impaired kidney, however, can neither excrete H^+ nor make extra HCO_3^- for buffering. The amount of HCO_3^- that exists is used up with the circulating acid. NH_4^+ excretion, another method for eliminating acid, is also decreased due to the lack of available ions (see Chapter 28). Because chronic renal failure is a slowly progressing disease, the body has time to compensate for the imbalance more easily than with an acute acidotic situation.

Electrolyte Disturbances

Potassium

Oliguria is responsible for causing hyperkalemia. Potassium is primarily excreted from the body via the kidneys, and when little to no urine output exists potassium is reabsorbed. In addition, due to the acidotic state, intracellular potassium is exchanged for the excess hydrogen ion, contributing more potassium to the elevated extracellular levels. The normal therapeutic range for potassium is 3.5–5.3 mEq/L. In renal failure levels may rise as high as 7.0 or 8.0 mEq/L, contributing to life-threatening cardiac dysrhythmias and cardiac arrest.

Question: Why does the serum potassium level increase with chronic renal failure?

Answer: Potassium is primarily excreted from the body via the kidneys, and when little to no urine output exists potassium is reabsorbed.

Calcium and Phosphate

In an azotemic state the gastrointestinal system cannot absorb calcium due to the lack of activated vitamin D normally created by the kidneys. This results in hypocalcemia. At the same time phosphate levels, normally cleared by the kidneys, rise because the kidneys are now functioning with a glomerular filtration rate below 25% of normal. Phosphate, inversely related to calcium, elevates as the calcium decreases. Due to the low calcium levels, the parathyroid hormone becomes activated and a resorption of calcium from bone takes place (see Chapter 17). At the expense of the skeletal system, calcium levels are maintained. Eventually, however, hyperparathyroidism occurs due to constant stimulation of the gland. A precipitation of calcium–phosphate salts eventually accumulates in the soft tissues of the body, particularly around joints, causing arthritic pain. Consequently, the patient must diligently adhere to a low-phosphate and low-protein diet.

Sodium

Initially, in chronic renal failure sodium is lost, causing an osmotic diuresis. This loss of water creates a dehydrated state. As oliguria occurs, sodium is retained along with water. This may contribute to a dilutional hyponatremia or, depending on the fluid balance, hypernatremic. A hypernatremic state may contribute to hypertension, edema, or congestive heart failure.

Magnesium

Magnesium, like other electrolytes, is excreted by the kidneys, and the patient with chronic renal failure is at risk for increased serum magnesium levels. If the patient follows a low-protein diet, decreased absorption of magnesium via the gastrointestinal tract helps to keep magnesium levels close to normal. In contrast, an increased intake of magnesium, such as with an overuse of antacids, can lead to a worsened state of hypermagnesium. All products containing magnesium should be avoided in chronic renal failure.

TREATMENT AND NURSING IMPLICATIONS

Neurological

Neurological changes occur as renal failure progresses; these changes often are an indication that dialysis should be initiated. Though the cause is not completely known, it is believed that the toxic accumulation of waste products and electrolyte imbalances contribute to an altered mentation. Assessment should include alertness, irritability, listlessness, or confusion. Observation for tetany, paresthesias, or muscle weakness should be conducted because these occurrences may be signs of an electrolyte imbalance.

Cardiovascular

Hypotension may develop if fluid loss occurs; however, hypertension is more common secondary to hypernatremia and fluid retention. Congestive heart failure may also result from the fluid overload or from left ventricular hypertrophy. If congestive heart failure occurs, basilar crackles and dyspnea may be present. Peripheral edema and distended neck veins may be present with fluid overload. A pericardial rub may be heard due to the pericarditis that develops from uremia. An irregular pulse may develop along with cardiac dysrhythmias from hyperkalemia. Monitoring vital signs and fluid and electrolyte balance are essential. Cardiac monitoring may be necessary if dysrhythmias develop. Antihypertensives, such as calcium channel blockers and angiotensin-converting enzyme inhibitors, may be needed if sodium and fluid restriction are not effective. Blood pressure needs to be adjusted carefully because the kidneys have been dependent on a hypertensive blood flow driven through atherosclerotic vessels.

Patients become anemic due to the decreased production of erythropoietin, a hormone produced by the kidneys responsible for stimulating red blood cell production. Additional factors contributing to the patient's anemic state include a decreased red blood cell life span; hemolysis due to excessive intake of sodium in the red blood cell, causing the cell to swell and burst; bleeding from the gastrointestinal tract; and frequent blood samples needed to monitor the client's condition. Hemoglobin and hematocrit levels should be monitored closely. Human erythropoietin may be available to treat the anemia.

Electrolyte

Potassium levels and the patient's cardiac status should be closely monitored. A potassium-restricted diet may be necessary. Diuretics or Kayexalate, a cation-exchange resin, may help to eliminate excess potassium. If necessary, dialysis will help to adjust the potassium to a normal level.

All electrolyte and, in particular, potassium levels should be closely monitored in chronic renal failure. Because of the decreased urine output, renal failure patients do not excrete enough potassium, and lethal dysrhythmias may develop. Diet should be evaluated for proper food choices.

Phosphate intake should be restricted, and if levels are excessive, calcium-based phosphate binders may be given. Calcium carbonate (Tums) or Amphojel may be used to help bind phosphate and elevate calcium levels. Antacids containing magnesium elevate the magnesium level, and patients should be cautioned about overuse of these products.

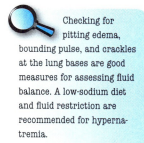

Checking for pitting edema, bounding pulse, and crackles at the lung bases are good measures for assessing fluid balance. A low-sodium diet and fluid restriction are recommended for hypernatremia.

Checking for pitting edema, bounding pulse, and crackles at the lung bases are good measures for assessing fluid balance. A low-sodium diet and fluid restriction are recommended for hypernatremia.

Respiratory

A predisposition to respiratory infections such as pneumonia or a uremic pleuritis develops. Pulmonary edema or dyspnea from fluid overload may occur and can be treated with diuretics or fluid removal with dialysis. Kussmaul respirations occur if the state of acidosis becomes severe. The patient should be assessed for shortness of breath and crackles, as well as for deep rapid respirations associated with acidosis.

Gastrointestinal

Mucosal ulcerations, bleeding, and stomatitis secondary to the bacterial breakdown of urea are common. Anorexia frequently accompanies gastrointestinal problems, contributing to nutritional deficiencies. Diarrhea may result from hyperkalemia. Calcium absorption is impaired. Complications associated with the gastrointestinal system are numerous and affect the patient's ability to eat and quality of life.

Protein restriction may help retard the degeneration of renal function. Adequate nutrition is important or the catabolism of proteins occurs. The breakdown of protein leads to increased urea, potassium, and phosphate levels; therefore a low-protein, high-caloric diet is needed for the patient not undergoing dialysis. A higher intake of protein is allowed if the patient is undergoing dialysis.

Question: What type of diet should be given to the chronic renal patient?

Answer: The breakdown of protein leads to increased urea, potassium, and phosphate levels; therefore a low-protein, high-caloric diet is needed for the patient not undergoing dialysis. A higher intake of protein is allowed if the patient is undergoing dialysis.

Musculoskeletal

Renal osteodystrophy may develop in relation to the alterations in calcium and phosphate balance. The metabolic acidosis, decreased synthesis of vitamin D, and calcium and phosphorus imbalances combine to create this faulty bone condition that results in spontaneous fractures. Each of these conditions treated separately, such as lowering the phosphate level, supplementing calcium, administering an active form of vitamin D, and attempting to correct the acidosis, can help to decrease the destruction of bone.

Integumentary

Dry skin along with calcium and phosphorus deposits on the skin can lead to a severe pruritus. When blood urea nitrogen levels elevate beyond normal, urea crystallizes on the skin, causing a condition known as uremic frost. Offering skin care with tepid water using nondrying soaps, applying creams, and administering antihistamines provide relief for the itching.

Drug Therapy

Medications must be administered cautiously to patients with chronic renal failure. Almost all drugs are excreted partially or completely through the renal system. Because renal clearance is decreased, toxicity is a concern. Drugs may need to be administered in decreased dosages or less frequently to allow for renal clearance.

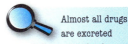 Almost all drugs are excreted partially or completely through the renal system. Because renal clearance is decreased, toxicity is a concern. Drugs may need to be administered in decreased dosages or less frequently to allow for renal clearance.

 Medications must be administered cautiously to patients with chronic renal failure.

Diabetes insipidus and syndrome of inappropriate diuretic hormone are two conditions of abnormal antidiuretic hormone secretion that affect fluid and electrolyte balance. In this chapter we discuss the clinical manifestations, treatment, and nursing implications for both conditions.

43

Disorders of Antidiuretic Hormone Regulation

TERMS
- ☐ **Antidiuretic hormone (ADH)**
- ☐ **Diabetes insipidus (DI)**
- ☐ **Syndrome of inappropriate diuretic hormone (SIADH)**

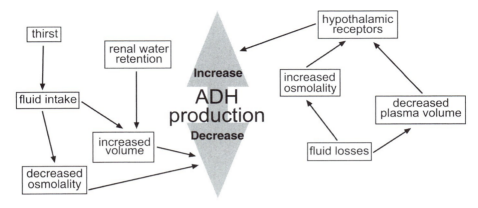

Figure 43-1 ADH production.

Antidiuretic hormone (ADH) is synthesized and regulated by the hypothalamus. When thirst occurs the body responds by increasing fluid intake and water retention. This helps to increase the volume of water in the body, decreasing osmolality and, therefore, decreasing ADH production. When the body loses an increased amount of fluid, decreasing plasma volume and increasing osmolality, the hypothalamic receptors increase ADH production to retain fluid and create a state of homeostasis (Figure 43-1).

Diabetes insipidus (DI) and **syndrome of inappropriate diuretic hormone (SIADH)** are two conditions of abnormal ADH secretion that affect fluid and electrolyte balance (Table 43-1). ADH is secreted by the hypothalamus to work on the renal tubules, increasing permeability for water and urea. When an insult to the cranium such as head trauma, tumors, or neurosurgery occurs, ADH secretion may be affected.

DIABETES INSIPIDUS

Two types of DI can occur: neurogenic and nephrogenic. Neurogenic DI is related to the lack of release of ADH, even when hypertonic solutions that increase the plasma osmolality are administered. Nephrogenic DI occurs when the renal system cannot respond to ADH even when pharmacological preparations of the hormone are administered.

Table 43-1 Disorders of Antidiuretic Hormone Production

DI	SIADH
↑ Urine output	↓ Urine output
↑ Osmolality/dehydration	↓ Osmolality/water gain
↑ Sodium	↓ Sodium (dilutional)
Polydipsia	Nausea/muscle cramps
Confusion/lethargy/coma	Anorexia/fatigue
	Seizures/coma

↑ Increased; ↓ decreased.

Clinical Manifestations

Patients with DI lack the ability to concentrate urine; consequently, they put out vast quantities, sometimes as much as 15 L/day of dilute urine. Polydipsia generally accompanies the high urine output; therefore, if the patient is capable, enough water can be consumed to maintain an adequate fluid balance.

Patients with DI lack the ability to concentrate urine; consequently, they put out vast quantities, sometimes as much as 15 L/day of dilute urine.

Dehydration problems occur when the output is extreme and the person is unable to maintain the intake to equal the urine output or if the patient is unconscious and unaware of the need for fluid. An increased serum osmolality and hypertonic dehydration occur. Hypernatremia exists with DI due to the loss of water without the loss of sodium. Symptoms of thirst and confusion may occur. If the condition goes undiagnosed, the symptoms may progress to lethargy and seizures.

Treatment

Management of DI includes treatment of any underlying cause, replacement of fluid, and administration of ADH preparations. Such preparations must be given by nasal insufflation because they are destroyed in the gastrointestinal tract if given orally.

Nursing Implications

Monitoring intravenous and oral fluid replacement is important. Measurement of intake and output along with daily weights are necessary. Serum electrolyte levels, especially sodium, must be closely monitored.

Monitoring of serum electrolyte levels, especially sodium, along with fluid volume is of vital importance in patients with DI.

SYNDROME OF INAPPROPRIATE ANTIDIURETIC HORMONE

SIADH occurs when the feedback loop for the release and inhibition of ADH malfunctions. Even when serum osmolality is low and urine output should be increased, ADH continues to be secreted, resulting in clinical manifestations of water intoxication.

Clinical Manifestations

A dilutional hyponatremia is present along with a serum hypoosmolality due to the abnormal reabsorption of water. Urine output decreases. Patients may complain of weight gain, headache, muscle cramps, anorexia, and fatigue related to the low sodium and excess water. If the condition persists with a sodium level of less than 125 mEq/L developing, nausea and vomiting may occur, leading to a greater electrolyte imbalance and seizures and coma.

 A severe sodium hyponatremia, secondary to SIADH, may result in nausea, vomiting, seizures, and coma. Electrolytes must be closely monitored.

Treatment

Fluid restriction is the treatment for mild cases. Diuretics may also be necessary to eliminate excess fluid gain. If the sodium level is quite low, hypertonic saline solutions, such as 3% NaCl, may be required.

Nursing Implications

Assessing the level of consciousness is helpful, especially when looking for signs of hyponatremia. Accurate intake and output measurement, along with daily weights, are of extreme importance. Laboratory values should be monitored for electrolyte imbalance.

Assessing the level of consciousness is helpful, especially when looking for signs of hyponatremia.

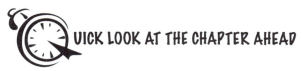

Respiratory failure occurs when the system is no longer able to exchange oxygen for carbon dioxide. Either a situation exists where sufficient oxygen is not available for transfer to the blood, resulting in hypoxemia, or carbon dioxide cannot be removed and is allowed to accumulate to dangerous levels, causing hypercapnia. In this chapter we examine hypoxemic and hypercapnic respiratory failure, the clinical manifestations, and treatment and nursing implications.

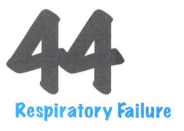

44

Respiratory Failure

TERMS
- [ ] **Hypercapnic respiratory failure**
- [ ] **Hypoventilation**
- [ ] **Intrapulmonary shunt**
- [ ] **Ventilation-perfusion (V/Q)**

CAUSES

Respiratory failure occurs when the system is no longer able to exchange oxygen for carbon dioxide. Either a situation exists where sufficient oxygen is not available for transfer to the blood, resulting in hypoxemia, or carbon dioxide cannot be removed and is allowed to accumulate to dangerous levels, causing hypercapnia. It is not a disease in itself but the result of a disease, respiratory or otherwise. Two types of respiratory failure exist, hypoxemic failure and hypercapnic failure.

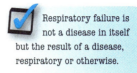
Respiratory failure is not a disease in itself but the result of a disease, respiratory or otherwise.

HYPOXEMIC FAILURE

Hypoxemia results from three different situations in the lung: alveolar hypoventilation, **ventilation-perfusion (V/Q) mismatch**, and an **intrapulmonary shunt** (Figure 44-1). As the term indicates, a lack or insufficient amount of oxygen exists in the blood for proper oxygenation. In hypoxemic failure the PaO_2 level falls below 60 mm Hg.

Alveolar Hypoventilation

Hypoventilation may be caused by a variety of conditions and results in decreased pO_2 and increased pCO_2 levels. Head injury or drug overdose

---

Alveolar Hypoventilation = ↓PaO_2 + ↑CO_2

V/Q Mismatch = Affected Ventilation + Unaffected Perfusion

OR

Affected Perfusion + Unaffected Ventilation

Shunt = Alveoli Filled with Fluid = No Gas Exchange

Figure 44-1 Hypoxemic failure.

may cause a decreased respiratory drive, leading to hypoventilation. Neuromuscular conditions exist that affect the respiratory muscles, such as amyotrophic lateral sclerosis or Guillain-Barré. Chest wall dysfunction associated with trauma or lung diseases, such as chronic obstructive pulmonary disease, cystic fibrosis, or acute respiratory distress syndrome, contribute to hypoventilation. Regardless of the cause, all affect the alveoli and gas exchange, causing hypoxemia.

V/Q Mismatch

V/Q mismatch refers to discrepancies in ventilation-perfusion relationships (Figure 44-2). Although it is not an actual 1:1 ratio of ventilation to perfusion, overall the ratio is close and varies slightly in certain areas of the lung. In situations of an accumulation of fluid in the alveoli such as pneumonia, asthma resulting in bronchospasm, or the collapse of

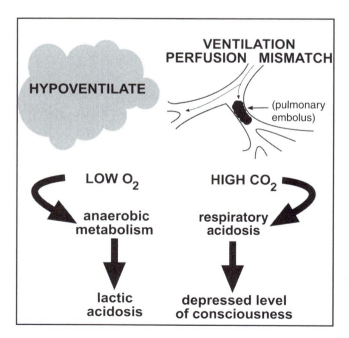

Figure 44-2   V/Q mismatch.

alveoli with atelectasis, air flow or ventilation is affected but perfusion to the alveoli continues unaffected. A pulmonary embolus is an example of the opposite. Because of the blockage of an embolus blood flow is interrupted, causing a perfusion problem, but ventilation continues unaffected. In such situations, regardless of whether ventilation or perfusion is affected, there is a mismatch.

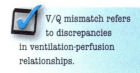

V/Q mismatch refers to discrepancies in ventilation-perfusion relationships.

Intrapulmonary Shunt

Unoxygenated blood exiting from the heart is generally the result of a shunt. A shunt can result from an anatomical abnormality such as a ventricular septal defect, where blood enters the right side of the heart then enters the left side of the heart through the septal defect without passing through the lungs. Another type of shunt is associated with pulmonary edema or acute respiratory distress syndrome. This type of shunt occurs when blood passes by alveoli that are filled with fluid and cannot participate with gas exchange. Some respiratory conditions, such as pneumonia or adult respiratory distress syndrome, may result in a combination of a V/Q mismatch and shunting.

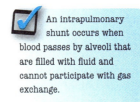

An intrapulmonary shunt occurs when blood passes by alveoli that are filled with fluid and cannot participate with gas exchange.

HYPERCAPNIC RESPIRATORY FAILURE

Hypercapnic respiratory failure is an inability to expel a sufficient amount of carbon dioxide, resulting in a failure in ventilation. Gas flow in and out of the lungs is normally adequate or exceeds the amount of ventilation needed to keep a normal $PaCO_2$ level. A person without lung disease has good ventilation at rest but is also able to exercise by increasing the need for maximum ventilation without suffering from an increased $PaCO_2$ level and respiratory failure. When demand exceeds supply for a person with lung disease, that person cannot expel the CO_2 and respiratory failure ensues. Hypercapnic failure is confirmed by arterial blood gas values with abnormally high $PaCO_2$ levels.

CLINICAL MANIFESTATIONS OF ACUTE RESPIRATORY FAILURE

When a lack of O_2 or an increase in CO_2 occurs acutely, an emergency situation exists. Failure to meet the oxygen needs of the tissues can result in a major insult to the body. Early manifestations are related to the central nervous system. Confusion, irritability, anxiety, and combative behavior are warning signs of hypoxemia. If the oxygen deprivation continues, the body shifts to an anaerobic (without oxygen) metabolism, which consumes more energy than an aerobic (with oxygen) metabolism. In addition, the waste product of anaerobic metabolism is lactic acid, which requires bicarbonate for buffering. If enough bicarbonate does not exist, such as with patients suffering from chronic renal failure, then metabolic acidosis occurs along with respiratory acidosis, resulting in a mixed disturbance (see Chapter 35). When the body is in a state of acidosis, the compensatory mechanism of exchanging H^+ for K^+ is initiated, contributing to a state of hyperkalemia (see Chapter 27).

Heart rate, respiratory rate, and cardiac output increase in an attempt to compensate for hypoxemia or to blow off CO_2. Accessory respiratory muscles are used, and the normal inspiratory-expiratory ratio of 1:2 is increased to 1:3 or 1:4 in an attempt to expel the CO_2. The workload to keep up this increase is difficult, especially if lactic acid, which develops in an anaerobic environment, is already present. Respiratory compromise occurs and failure ensues.

Respiratory alkalosis may occur from hyperventilation and an excess loss of carbon dioxide. If this occurs, the exchange of H^+ for K^+ reverses, with H^+ exiting the cell and K^+ entering the cell, causing a potential hypokalemia in the extracellular fluid, depending on the severity of the alkalosis.

TREATMENT AND NURSING IMPLICATIONS

Supplemental oxygen therapy is helpful for patients with a V/Q mismatch because not all areas of the lung are affected and additional oxygen is needed to compensate for the mismatched areas. Patients suffering from alveolar hypoventilation or a shunt problem do not benefit as easily from supplemental oxygen because of the fluid-filled alveoli that are unable to participate in gas exchange. Mechanical ventilation may be required for this type of patient with the addition of positive end-expiratory pressure to help inflate the alveoli. Proper suctioning and maintenance of ventilator settings assist the patient's respiratory status. The type of oxygen management depends on the condition causing the hypoxemia or hypercapnia. Arterial blood gas and electrolyte levels should be monitored closely.

> A patient with a shunt should be placed on a ventilator with positive end-expiratory pressure. Positive end-expiratory pressure is the application of positive pressure during exhalation to help lung volume during exhalation to remain greater than normal.

Assessing the patient neurologically for hypoxic manifestations is important for early intervention. As the condition worsens, the patient's level of consciousness may become depressed. Respiratory assessment should include auscultation for air exchange in all lung fields, observation of accessory muscle use, and rate, depth, and character of respirations. Hemodynamic monitoring to assess blood flow and oxygenation is essential as well as monitoring laboratory values and arterial blood gas values. Cardiac monitoring is important for evaluation of dysrhythmias related to electrolyte imbalance and respiratory depression. Administering bronchodilators and corticosteroids is helpful in opening the airways and decreasing swelling. Fluid balance should also be maintained.

As a condition worsens, a patient's level of consciousness may become depressed; therefore assessing the patient neurologically for hypoxic manifestations is important for early intervention to take place.

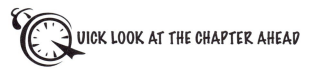

Pulmonary edema can result from numerous noncardiogenic causes affecting the lung. In this chapter we discuss fluid balance and gas exchange in the lung along with clinical manifestations, treatment, and nursing implications for noncardiogenic causes of pulmonary edema.

45

Noncardiogenic Pulmonary Edema

TERMS
☐ **Pulmonary edema**

CAUSES

The source for pulmonary edema is frequently a failing cardiac system. **Pulmonary edema**, however, can result from numerous causes affecting the lung. Situations involving alveolar damage such as septicemia, inhalation injuries with smoke or poisonous gases, or aspiration of toxic fluids can cause increased capillary permeability in the lung bed. Drug-induced injury from chemotherapeutic agents, heroin, and inhalants can also be the source of pulmonary edema. Other situations involving high altitude, head injury, lymphatic obstruction associated with malignant processes, or decreased colloidal osmotic pressure associated with liver or other wasting diseases can all be considered causes of noncardiogenic pulmonary edema (Figure 45-1).

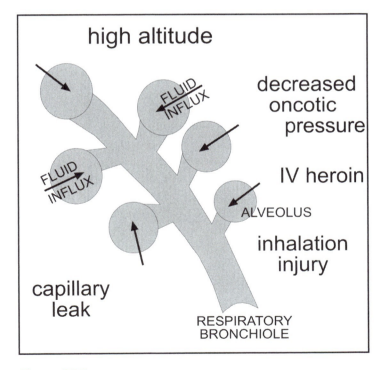

Figure 45-1 Causes of noncardiogenic pulmonary edema.

PATHOPHYSIOLOGY

The primary function of the pulmonary circulation is to facilitate gas exchange. The pulmonary circulatory system has low resistance and low pressure. In comparison with the systemic circulation with an arterial

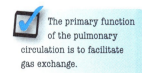

The primary function of the pulmonary circulation is to facilitate gas exchange.

mean pressure of 90 mm Hg, the mean pressure of the pulmonary artery is 15 mm Hg. This low pressure allows for greater increases in pulmonary blood flow during exercise and for the workload of the right ventricle to be less than that of the left ventricle.

FLUID BALANCE

In the normal lung a balance exists between the hydrostatic and oncotic pressures in the capillary beds. This balance prevents fluid from leaking out of the capillary (see Chapter 7). If, however, the hydrostatic pressure increases or the colloidal oncotic pressure decreases, an interstitial pulmonary edema develops from the fluid leaving the capillaries and entering the interstitium. Initially, the lymphatic system helps to transport excess

The exchange of gases in the lung involves the movement of oxygen from the alveoli to the capillary and carbon dioxide from the capillary to the alveoli. Once fluid begins to enter the alveoli, gas exchange becomes impaired.

fluid; however, as fluid continues to leave the pulmonary capillaries, excessive amounts begin to overwhelm the system, causing the fluid to push into the alveoli, resulting in pulmonary edema. This becomes detrimental to one's ability to breathe. Once fluid begins to enter the alveoli, gas exchange becomes impaired.

GAS EXCHANGE

Oxygen and carbon dioxide are exchanged by diffusion, from an area of higher concentration to an area of lower concentration, in the pulmonary bed. The gases diffuse easily across the alveolar and capillary walls because these walls are only one cell thick. The exchange involves the movement of oxygen from the alveoli to the capillary and carbon dioxide

Table 45-1 Noncardiogenic Pulmonary Edema Clinical Manifestations

Feeling of impending doom
Restlessness/agitation
Dyspnea
Tachypnea
Dry cough leading to frothy, blood-tinged sputum
Respiratory acidosis
Bilateral crackles at lung bases

from the capillary to the alveoli. The oxygen-rich blood is then circulated to the heart and eventually the tissues, whereas the carbon dioxide is removed from the alveoli during expiration. In pulmonary edema the alveoli are filled with fluid and cannot contribute to the exchange of gases. Carbon dioxide levels increase and oxygen levels decrease.

CLINICAL MANIFESTATIONS

Dyspnea and tachypnea develop as the alveoli fill with fluid (Table 45-1). The patient complains of a "lack of air" and a "feeling of impending doom." A cough develops with sputum that becomes frothy and blood tinged. Crackles are audible at the bases of the lungs. Arterial blood gas results will indicate a respiratory acidosis, decreased PaO_2, and increased pCO_2 as the condition worsens.

TREATMENT AND NURSING IMPLICATIONS

Oxygen administration is most important. Diuretics must be given to alleviate the excess fluids. Fluid and electrolyte balance must be maintained, and any imbalances must be corrected. At times, mechanical ventilation with positive end-expiratory pressure is required to provide additional respiratory support. Identification of the underlying cause is necessary to determine the remaining treatment.

Oxygen administration and diuretic therapy is essential for patients suffering from noncardiogenic pulmonary edema. When diuretics are given, fluid and electrolyte balance must be closely monitored.

 QUICK LOOK AT THE CHAPTER AHEAD

Heart failure is an abnormal condition of the heart's ability to pump blood to meet the metabolic needs of the tissues and results from multiple health problems or risk factors. In this chapter we look at the pathology of heart failure and the severe clinical manifestations that result from it. Treatment and nursing implications are also discussed.

46

Heart Failure

TERMS
- [ ] **Cor pulmonale**
- [ ] **Diastolic failure**
- [ ] **Dyspnea**
- [ ] **Heart failure**
- [ ] **Left-sided cardiac failure**
- [ ] **Left ventricular ejection failure**
- [ ] **Orthopnea**
- [ ] **Paroxysmal nocturnal dyspnea**
- [ ] **Systolic failure**

CAUSES OF HEART FAILURE

Heart failure is an abnormal condition of the heart's ability to pump blood to meet the metabolic needs of the tissues. Heart failure results from multiple health problems or risk factors, including obesity and elevated cholesterol levels, that lead to coronary artery disease. Long-term diabetes mellitus causes severe damage to the vascular system and causes a predisposition to heart failure. Heart failure frequently occurs secondary to damaged cardiac muscle. Myocardial infarction, ventricular aneurysm, and myocarditis are problems that affect the contractility of the heart. Ventricular overload, which is the result of increased blood return to the heart, may also result in congestive heart failure. Most commonly, heart failure results from hypertension associated with atherosclerosis of the heart and blood vessels from sustained elevated high blood pressure levels. Whatever the cause, heart failure results in an increased workload for the ventricles. The increased workload of the heart eventually causes both the right and left ventricles to fail and improperly supply the body with oxygenated blood.

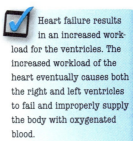

Heart failure results in an increased workload for the ventricles. The increased workload of the heart eventually causes both the right and left ventricles to fail and improperly supply the body with oxygenated blood.

Numerous terms have been used to further describe heart failure, including forward and backward heart failure, low- and high-output failure, systolic and diastolic dysfunction (Figure 46-1), right-sided and left-sided failure, or congestive heart failure, a more precise term when circulatory or pulmonary congestion is present. Currently, systolic and diastolic and right-sided and left-sided are the commonly used terms to describe heart failure. Regardless of the description used to identify heart failure, as the disease progresses into a chronic condition the terms no longer seem different and tend to blend together. Emerging symptoms and system deterioration ultimately lead to a diminished quality of life and shortened life expectancy.

PATHOLOGY

Systolic Failure

Systolic failure occurs when the left ventricle (systolic function) is affected by an event that affects the contractility of the cardiac muscle fibers, making the left ventricle unable to pump the blood effectively and

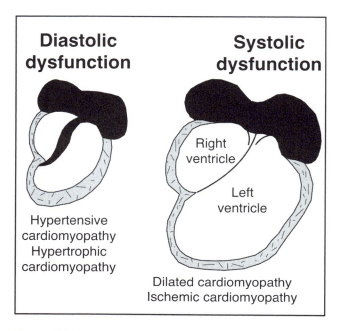

Figure 46-1 Diastolic and systolic dysfunction.

empty completely. Attempts to pump blood from the left ventricle against the high pressured aorta fail, decreasing the **left ventricular ejection fraction** (the amount of blood ejected from the heart per beat, taking into consideration the entire amount of blood available per beat) and leaving blood in the ventricle, which increases the left ventricular end-diastolic pressure. During subsequent cardiac cycles, the regular amount of blood is propelled from the right ventricle to the lungs to the left atrium and into the left ventricle. Already filled with blood from the previous cycle, the left ventricle cannot accept the quantity prepared for it. Eventually, blood accumulates in the pulmonary circulation, elevating the pulmonary capillary wedge pressure. Systolic failure is associated with dilated cardiomyopathy and ischemic cardiomyopathy, along with other disorders.

Diastolic Failure

Diastolic failure occurs when the ventricles become unable to sufficiently relax and fill completely (diastolic function), resulting in a decreased amount of oxygenated blood returning from the lungs to the heart. Diastole is the heart's time to rest and passively fill with blood. Systole occurs when the heart contracts to pump blood to the tissues. In diastolic failure the ventricles become stiff and noncompliant. Though the cardiac contraction may be effective, the high filling pressures and venous engorgement of the pulmonary and systemic vascular systems that the ventricles must pump against result in a noncompliant ventricle that does not fill properly. Diastolic failure occurs secondary to left ventricular hypertrophy, systemic hypertension, or aortic stenosis.

Left-Sided Failure

Left- and right-sided failure refer to the side of the heart with the initial impairment. **Left-sided cardiac failure** results when the heart can no longer pump a sufficient amount of blood to supply the tissues, causing blood to back up into the left atrium and pulmonary veins. Many conditions cause the left side of the heart to fail. Hypertension and myocardial infarction are two examples. Hypertension forces the ventricle to continuously pump against high pressures. This eventually leads to a hypertrophied muscle with poor contractility. Myocardial infarctions result in scar tissue that causes that particular area of the ventricular wall to lose elasticity and contractility. Both hypertension and myocardial infarction result in left-sided failure. Dyspnea, **orthopnea** (shortness of breath in a recumbent position), **paroxysmal nocturnal dyspnea** (sudden intermittent spasms of difficult breathing occurring at night), and a dry hacking cough (initially) are symptoms that accompany the pulmonary edema (Table 46-1).

Right-Sided Failure

Because the right side of the heart works with the left, right-sided failure generally results from left-sided problems; however, other conditions

Table 46-1 Symptoms of Left-Sided Heart Failure

Fatigue
Pulmonary congestion
Pulmonary edema
Dyspnea
Orthopnea
Paroxysmal nocturnal dyspnea

Table 46-2 Symptoms of Right-Sided Heart Failure

Fatigue
Jugular vein distension
Peripheral edema (e.g., extremities, sacrum)
Right upper quadrant pain (e.g., hepatomegaly, splenomegaly)
Gastrointestinal bloating (ascites, nausea)

such as **cor pulmonale** (right ventricular enlargement secondary to lung disease), right ventricular infarction, or chronic pulmonary hypertension also contribute to right-sided failure. With blood backing up into the pulmonary bed, the right ventricle pumps harder to propel blood into the pulmonary artery. Eventually, the right ventricle fatigues after the left ventricle. Blood backs up into the systemic venous circulation, causing jugular venous distension, peripheral edema, and vascular congestion of the gastrointestinal tract, including the liver and spleen (Table 46-2).

CLINICAL MANIFESTATIONS

Dyspnea

Dyspnea, difficulty breathing, is a common sign in heart failure. In the early stages it occurs with activity. As the disease becomes progressively worse, dyspnea occurs more readily with less strenuous activities, eventually occurring at rest. Cardiac dyspnea is recognized in patients suffering from an engorged pulmonary vasculature and pulmonary interstitial edema, which affects lung compliance. When lung compliance is affected, the workload of the accessory muscles used to inflate the lungs increases. Breathing becomes more rapid and shallow, affecting the delivery of oxygen to these overworked muscles. Coupled with a decreased cardiac output, the shortness of breath contributes to fatigue, keeping the patient's activity at a minimum. Oxygen therapy becomes a fact of life along with restricted activity. Diuretics may be helpful with fluid overload.

Pulmonary Edema

Pulmonary edema occurs when the alveoli of the lungs fill with serosanguineous fluid. This situation can be a life-threatening manifestation of congestive heart failure. The patient may be agitated due to decreased oxygenation. Dyspnea, the use of accessory respiratory muscles, and an increased respiratory rate are common. Crackles and wheezes may be heard on auscultation, and the patient may produce blood-tinged and frothy sputum. The patient may appear cyanotic, and the skin becomes cool and clammy as vasoconstriction occurs in an attempt to keep the vital organs perfused. Tachycardia develops due to stimulation of the sympathetic nervous system sensing a decreased cardiac output. The blood pressure either elevates or decreases depending on the severity of the edema and ability of the heart to maintain an increased rate.

This condition requires immediate attention. Oxygen should be administered. Aggressive treatment with loop diuretics such as furosemide, administered intravenously, and fluid restriction are necessary. Morphine sulfate helps to decrease the left ventricular end-diastolic pressure and to alleviate the patient's anxiety and feelings of impending doom. Inotropic drugs help to increase cardiac output and decrease the increased systemic vascular resistance.

 Pulmonary edema can be a life-threatening condition requiring immediate treatment with oxygen, diuretics, MSO$_4$, and inotropic drugs.

Peripheral Edema

Peripheral edema results from a local or generalized accumulation of fluid in the tissues. The lower extremities or sacrum of the patient if sedentary or bedridden may be edematous, the liver may become engorged (hepatomegaly), the abdomen may retain fluid (ascites), or the spleen may retain fluid (splenomegaly). Diuretics help to alleviate the excess fluid along with fluid restriction.

Electrolyte Imbalances

Hyponatremia may result from a dilutional affect or from overaggressive diuretic therapy. Hypomagnesemia may also occur with heavy diuretic use. Hypokalemia results from excessive diuretic use, but hyperkalemia may occur from an acidotic state. Any electrolyte imbalance may lead to dysrhythmias in an already stressed and compromised heart.

Question: **What type of electrolyte imbalances might occur with the use of diuretics?**

Answer: **Hyponatremia, hypomagnesemia, or hypokalemia.**

Acid–Base Imbalance

Lactic acid, a product of anaerobic metabolism, is produced secondary to poor tissue perfusion. As lactic acid accumulates, metabolic acidosis occurs. In an attempt to compensate, the patient's respiratory rate increases to blow off CO_2, potentially resulting in a respiratory alkalosis. If the condition continues to the point of respiratory fatigue, carbon dioxide accumulates, causing a mixed disturbance of metabolic and respiratory acidosis.

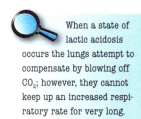 When a state of lactic acidosis occurs the lungs attempt to compensate by blowing off CO_2; however, they cannot keep up an increased respiratory rate for very long.

TREATMENT

Oxygen is a priority in the treatment of heart failure. Pulse oximetry monitoring, if the patient is hospitalized, to determine oxygen saturation is important along with the administration of oxygen. Diuretics such as the loop diuretic, furosemide, should be administered to help mobilize edematous fluid and reduce preload (ventricular filling pressure and the amount of stretch placed on the myocardial fibers). Potassium-sparing diuretics, such as spironolactone, may be used in combination with the loop diuretics. Vasodilators are also needed to reduce preload and afterload (the amount of peripheral resistance against which the left ventricle must pump), and inotropic agents are required to help strengthen the contractility of the heart. Morphine sulfate is frequently used to help decrease preload and afterload and for the additional benefit of decreasing anxiety. The beta-blocking drugs are also helpful for blocking the sympathetic nervous system adverse effect of an increased heart rate. A low-sodium diet (usually 2 g/day) is important to help minimize fluid retention.

It is important to monitor the patient's oxygen saturation with pulse oximetry when administering oxygen. Patients exhibiting restlessness, agitation, fatigue, or activity intolerance may be oxygen deprived.

NURSING IMPLICATIONS

Signs of congestive heart failure should be assessed and include agitation, fatigue, activity intolerance, and restlessness due to decreased oxygenation. Monitor vital signs and oxygen saturation, assess for a rapid respiratory rate, dyspnea, and cough related to the accumulation of fluid in the lungs. Auscultate the lung fields for crackles. Evaluate arterial blood gases for acid–base balance. Note edema that may be present in the lower extremities. Cardiac monitoring is important for identification of dysrhythmias that may develop secondary to an imbalance of sodium and potassium electrolyte levels. Administer oxygen and medications as ordered.

QUICK LOOK AT THE CHAPTER AHEAD

Diabetic ketoacidosis (DKA) is a serious complication of diabetes mellitus where the patient manifests a blood glucose > 250 mg/dL, serum pH < 7.3, serum HCO_3 < 15 mEq/L, and ketonemia or ketonuria. DKA results from too little insulin in relation to an increased caloric intake or increased bodily stress. In this chapter we identify how DKA occurs, the clinical manifestations, and treatment and nursing implications.

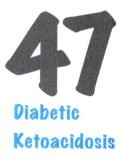

47

Diabetic Ketoacidosis

TERMS
- ☐ **Diabetes mellitus**
- ☐ **Diabetic ketoacidosis (DKA)**

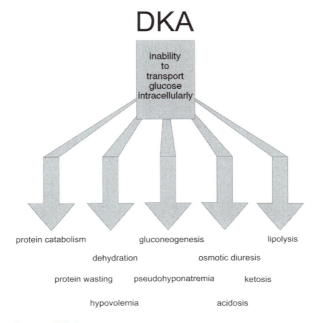

Figure 47-1 Diabetic ketoacidosis.

Diabetes mellitus is a group of heterogeneous disorders that affect carbohydrate metabolism and glucose homeostasis. There are two classifications of diabetes: type 1, characterized by pancreatic B-cell destruction requiring insulin replacement, and type 2, characterized by a secretory defect in insulin production and a resistance to the action of insulin on peripheral tissues. Type 2 diabetes can be controlled with diet and exercise. Under normal conditions, insulin is released into the bloodstream continuously and increases with demands such as snacks and meals. Acute and chronic complications can happen with abnormal insulin release. Hyperglycemia and hypoglycemia are two extremes of blood glucose imbalance. **Diabetic ketoacidosis (DKA)**, discussed in this chapter, and hyperosmolar hyperglycemic nonketotic syndrome, discussed in Chapter 48, are two critical hyperglycemic states.

DKA is a serious complication of diabetes mellitus where the patient manifests a blood glucose > 250 mg/dL, serum pH < 7.3, serum HCO_3 < 15 mEq/L, and ketonemia or ketonuria. DKA results from too little insulin in relation to an increased caloric intake or increased bodily stress. It primarily occurs with type 1 diabetes but can also take place with type 2 diabetes during times of severe illness or trauma that cause an increased demand for insulin that cannot be met. When insufficient insulin is not available for glucose metabolism or carbohydrate metabolism, the liver metabolizes fats (lipolysis) to supply the body's energy needs. Ketoacids are the product of this fat metabolism, and large quantities are released when carbohydrate stores are limited or cannot be accessed. An increased H^+ load develops as more ketones are produced than can be used, resulting in metabolic acidosis. With an altered pH, the body attempts to eliminate the ketones via urine, resulting in ketonuria. In an attempt to correct the state of acidosis, buffering cations, such as bicarbonate and potassium, are depleted with the excretion of ketoacids, and the acidotic state worsens.

Diabetic keto-acidosis results from too little insulin in relation to an increased caloric intake or increased bodily stress. When sufficient insulin is not available for glucose metabolism or carbohydrate metabolism, the liver metabolizes fats (lipolysis) to supply the body's energy needs. Ketoacids are the product of this fat metabolism, and large quantities are released when carbohydrate stores are limited or cannot be accessed.

The body continues to need energy and as a compensatory mechanism generates glucose (gluconeogenesis) from the breakdown of protein. This results in a surplus of nitrogen and glucose that cannot be used because of the insufficient insulin levels. The plasma osmolality increases secondary to the increased state of hyperglycemia. This situation promotes the movement of intracellular fluid to the extracellular compartment, producing an osmotic diuresis. The increased loss of water contributes to a state of dehydration and electrolyte imbalances of potassium and sodium. In a state of acidosis, potassium is shifted from the intracellular compartment to the extracellular compartment in exchange for the hydrogen ion, contributing to the lowering of potassium levels. A pseudohyponatremia may occur along with the intracellular–extracellular fluid shift as water shifts to the extracellular compartment.

CLINICAL MANIFESTATIONS

Clinical manifestations of diabetic ketoacidosis are related to the inability to use glucose for energy, resulting in fatigue and irritability (Table 47-1). The blood glucose levels are greater than 250 mg/dL (normal fasting glu-

Table 47-1 Clinical Manifestations of DKA

Blood glucose levels > 250 mg/dL
Metabolic acidosis
Fatigue
Irritability
Kussmaul respirations
Fruity "acetone" breath
Flushed/dry skin
Dry mucous membranes
Increased thirst
Urinary frequency
    Glucosuria/ketonuria
Nausea/vomiting
    Acid–base imbalance
    Electrolyte loss
    Dehydration
        Hypotension
        Tachycardia

cose levels are 80–90 mg/dL), and the state of acidosis is manifested by a low pH (< 7.3) and a low bicarbonate level (< 15 mEq/L). Rapid and deep respirations (Kussmaul respirations) occur in an attempt to rid the body of excess acid by eliminating CO_2. One of the hallmark signs is a fruity or "acetone" breath that results from the excess ketones in the body. The skin becomes flushed and dry along with dry mucous membranes due to the dehydration. In the early stages patients develop an increased thirst. If vomiting occurs, dehydration, acid–base balance, and electrolyte loss are compounded. Hypotension and a weak rapid pulse also develop because of the low fluid volume and electrolyte imbalance. If left untreated, depression of the central nervous system leads to shock and coma.

Hypotension and a weak rapid pulse may develop because of low fluid volume and electrolyte imbalance. If left untreated, depression of the central nervous system leads to shock and coma.

TREATMENT AND NURSING IMPLICATIONS

Treatment of DKA involves correcting the fluid status, electrolyte imbalance, and acidosis. Fluid and electrolyte replacement is supplemented with intravenous solutions and based on plasma values. Most commonly, an intravenous solution of 0.45% or 0.9% NaCl is recommended to run at a rate of 1 L/hr until the blood pressure is stabilized and the urine output increases to 30–60 cc/hr. A bolus of short-acting insulin followed by continuous intravenous infusion of 0.1 U/kg/hr helps to stabilize the hyperglycemia and ketoacidosis. Care must be taken to gradually decrease the glucose levels. Once the blood glucose level approaches 250 mg/dL, dextrose is added to the intravenous solution to prevent the possibility of hypoglycemia. In the state of acidosis potassium levels elevate as

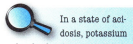

In a state of acidosis, potassium levels elevate as potassium flows into the extracellular compartment in exchange for the hydrogen ion, which moves into the cell. Therefore potassium levels may initially appear to be elevated; however, insulin drives potassium back into the cell, and as the acidosis is corrected potassium may need to be administered to correct any potential hypokalemic situations.

potassium flows into the extracellular compartment in exchange for the hydrogen ion, which moves into the cell. Therefore the potassium levels may initially appear to be elevated; however, insulin drives potassium back into the cell, and as the acidosis is corrected potassium may need to be administered to correct any potential hypokalemic situations. Careful monitoring of the patient's neurological status, vital signs, cardiac status, laboratory values, and intake and output are essential.

QUICK LOOK AT THE CHAPTER AHEAD

Hyperglycemic hyperosmolar nonketotic (HHNK) syndrome is a medical emergency that primarily affects patients with type 2 diabetes who can produce enough insulin to keep them from a state of acidosis but not enough to counteract the accumulation of excess glucose and the complicating high osmolarity and extracellular fluid loss. This syndrome is manifested by a blood sugar usually greater than 600 mg/dL and plasma osmolarity of 310 mOsm/L. In this chapter we review the causes and clinical manifestations of HHNK syndrome along with treatment and nursing implications.

48

Hyperglycemic Hyperosmolar Nonketotic Syndrome

TERMS
☐ Hyperglycemic hyperosmolar nonketotic (HHNK) syndrome

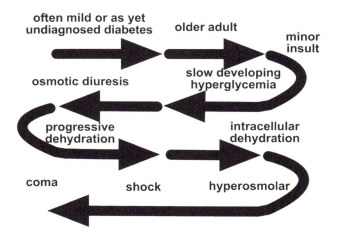

often mild or as yet undiagnosed diabetes

older adult

minor insult

slow developing hyperglycemia

osmotic diuresis

progressive dehydration

intracellular dehydration

coma

shock

hyperosmolar

Figure 48-1 Hyperglycemic hyperosmolar nonketotic syndrome.

CAUSES

Hyperglycemic hyperosmolar nonketotic (HHNK) syndrome is a complication of diabetes that primarily affects patients with type 2 diabetes. It is a medical emergency that affects individuals who can produce enough insulin to keep them from a state of acidosis but not enough to counteract the accumulation of excess glucose and the

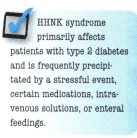

HHNK syndrome primarily affects patients with type 2 diabetes and is frequently precipitated by a stressful event, certain medications, intravenous solutions, or enteral feedings.

complicating high osmolarity and extracellular fluid loss. This event is frequently precipitated by a stressful event such as infection, trauma, myocardial infarction, thrombolytic events, or acute pancreatitis. It also has been associated with certain medications, such as phenytoin and thiazide diuretics, and procedures, such as peritoneal dialysis. Intravenous solutions containing a high glucose content, such as hyperalimentation or enteral feedings, have also been documented as precipitating HHNK syndrome. Older patients with a history of type 2 diabetes present with HHNK syndrome along with a recent history of polyuria and inadequate fluid intake.

CLINICAL MANIFESTATIONS

This syndrome is manifested by a blood sugar usually greater than 600 mg/dL and plasma osmolarity of 310 mOsm/L (Table 48-1). The elevated glucose draws fluid from the cell to the extracellular compartment, resulting in dehydration and causing dry mucous membranes, decreased skin turgor, and orthostatic hypotension. In addition, the

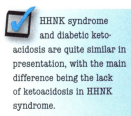

HHNK syndrome and diabetic keto-acidosis are quite similar in presentation, with the main difference being the lack of ketoacidosis in HHNK syndrome.

dehydration, if left untreated, affects the central nervous system, causing a somnolence and eventual coma and death. HHNK syndrome and diabetic ketoacidosis are quite similar in presentation, with the main difference being the lack of ketoacidosis in HHNK syndrome.

TREATMENT AND NURSING IMPLICATIONS

This condition is a medical emergency and carries a high mortality rate of approximately 50%. Treatment centers on restoring fluid balance from

Table 48-1 Clinical Manifestations of HHNK Syndrome

Blood glucose levels > 600 mg/dL
No acidosis
Plasma osmolarity of 310 mOsm/L
Dehydration
    Dry mucous membranes
    Decreased skin turgor
    Orthostatic hypotension
Somnolence, weakness, lethargy
Left untreated
    Coma
    Death

the high osmolar state to one of normalcy. Isotonic or hypotonic saline solutions are used for restoration; however, caution must be exercised to not administer fluids too aggressively, because of the risk of causing cerebral edema due to a sudden rehydration of previously dehydrated brain cells. A guideline is to replace one-half of the estimated fluid deficit in the first 12 hours.

Neurological assessment is an ongoing process, and measuring intake and output is extremely important. The patient's cardiac status should be monitored for dysrhythmias caused by the electrolyte imbalance. Electrolytes lost through the osmotic diuresis, especially sodium and potassium, must be replaced. Potassium also moves into the cell with the administration of insulin, compounding any state of hypokalemia that might exist.

Frequent measurement of blood glucose results should be conducted and short-acting insulin administered as a bolus followed by continuous intravenous infusion of 0.1 U/kg/hr to decrease the high blood glucose. Once the blood glucose has dropped to approximately 250 mg/dL, dextrose is added to the intravenous solution to prevent hypoglycemia. The underlying cause that triggered the event needs to be determined, along with educating the patient to prevent the event from happening in the future.

Isotonic or hypotonic saline solutions are used for restoration; however, caution must be exercised to not administer fluids too aggressively, because of the risk of causing cerebral edema due to a sudden rehydration of previously dehydrated brain cells.

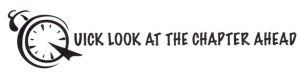

QUICK LOOK AT THE CHAPTER AHEAD

The physiological changes accompanying burn injury depend on the degree and surface area of the burn. Burns range from first-degree minor injuries that destroy the outermost layer of the epidermis to fourth-degree predominately fatal injuries involving muscle and bone.

49

Burns

TERMS

- ☐ First-degree burns
- ☐ Second-degree burns
- ☐ Third-degree burns
- ☐ Fourth-degree burns

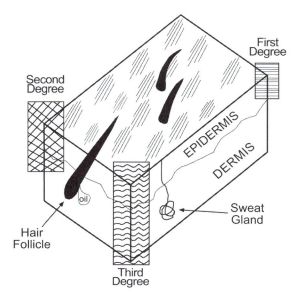

Figure 49-1 Burns.

The degree and surface area of burns determine the physiological changes that are seen. They range from first-degree minor injuries to fourth-degree predominately fatal injuries.

FIRST-DEGREE BURNS

First-degree injuries destroy the outermost layer of the epidermis but the skin remains intact. Blisters do not form, but erythema is present and the injured area is uncomfortable. **First-degree burns** occur from ultraviolet light exposure such as sunburn or a brief exposure to hot liquid. Aspirin or acetaminophen helps to relieve the discomfort.

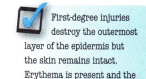

First-degree injuries destroy the outermost layer of the epidermis but the skin remains intact. Erythema is present and the injured area is uncomfortable.

Second-Degree Burns

Second-degree burns involve a partial-thickness injury to the tissue and are classified as superficial or deep. The superficial second-degree burn takes 3–4 weeks for proper healing, whereas the second-degree deep injury takes at least 30 or more days for complete healing.

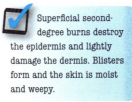

Superficial second-degree burns destroy the epidermis and lightly damage the dermis. Blisters form and the skin is moist and weepy.

Superficial second-degree burns destroy the epidermis and lightly damage the dermis. Blisters form and the skin appears to be moist and weepy. This type of injury may be caused by a brief exposure to flame or hot liquids. Pain sensors remain intact; therefore this type of burn is more painful than first-degree injuries. Generally, the site heals in 3 to 4 weeks provided infection does not occur.

Deep second-degree burns destroy the epidermis, dermis, and epidermal appendages. Blisters form but do not have the normal fluid-filled appearance. Instead, they are thin and paper-like. The injured area is mottled, waxy-white, pink, or red in color. This type of burn results from flame or scalding liquids. With deep tissue destruction pain sensors are destroyed; however, the area is surrounded by pain sensors in less damaged areas that are extremely sensitive to the injury. In healthy people and without the complication of infection, this type of injury heals in approximately 30 days. Skin grafting may be required.

With deep tissue destruction pain sensors are destroyed; however, the area is surrounded by pain sensors in less damaged areas that are extremely sensitive to the injury.

THIRD-DEGREE BURNS

Full-thickness **third-degree burns** destroy the epidermis, dermis, and epidermal appendages. Damage extends to the entire dermis, including the underlying subcutaneous tissue. The area of injury is dry and leather-like because of the loss of skin elasticity. The color is a mottled brown or red. Edema is present and combined with the leather-like skin can constrict the tissue like a tourniquet. Unless an escharotomy is performed to relieve the pressure, the skin will burst or all circulation will be lost to the area. This type of injury occurs with prolonged contact with flame, scalding liquids, or steam. It may also result from electrical current or

Full-thickness third-degree burns destroy the epidermis, entire dermis, and epidermal appendages. The area of injury is dry and leather-like because of the loss of skin elasticity. The color is a mottled brown or red.

direct contact with chemicals. The pain receptors of the injured area are destroyed, but, as with second-degree burns, there may be surrounding areas not as deeply burned that remain quite sensitive to pain. Skin grafting is required.

 With third-degree burns edema is present and combined with the leather-like skin can constrict the tissue like a tourniquet. Unless an escharotomy is performed to relieve the pressure, the skin will burst or all circulation will be lost to the area.

FOURTH-DEGREE BURNS

Fourth-degree burns are extremely serious injuries involving muscle and bone. The wound is dry and charred and mottled brown, white, or red in color. There is no sensation to pain except for surrounding tissues that may have a lesser burned area such as second- or third-degree burns. These

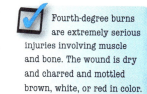

Fourth-degree burns are extremely serious injuries involving muscle and bone. The wound is dry and charred and mottled brown, white, or red in color.

injuries occur from contact with an electrical current or prolonged contact with flame. Skin grafting is required, and the limb may need to be amputated.

CLINICAL MANIFESTATIONS

Serious burn injuries can initially result in hypovolemic shock leading to hypoperfusion, acid–base and electrolyte imbalance, fluid loss, and organ failure. Initially, the increase in capillary endothelial permeability causes a massive shift of fluid from the vasculature. Sodium, water, and protein leak into the interstitial space, causing massive edema. As protein shifts from the vasculature to the interstitium, the colloidal osmotic pressure decreases, causing more fluid to shift (Figure 49-2). Second and third spacing take place as mediators of inflammation are released, causing vasodilation and compounding the hypotensive effect. As the circulating volume decreases, the blood pressure and cardiac output decrease. The compensatory sympathetic nervous system mechanisms take over,

Burn Injury
↓
↑Vascular Permeability = Edema + Protein Shift = ↓ Colloidal Osmotic Pressure
+
Loss of Skin Barrier = Evaporation
↓
↓ Circulating Volume = ↓ Blood Pressure and ↓ Cardiac Output
↓
↑Sympathetic Nervous System Stimulation = Vasoconstriction = ↑ Heart Rate and
↑ Cardiac Output

Figure 49-2 Clinical manifestations from burns.

producing vasoconstriction via renin-angiotensin activation and antidiuretic hormone secretion (see Chapter 8). The heart rate accelerates in an attempt to increase cardiac output. In addition to the fluid shifts, evaporation occurs through the lost skin barrier, also contributing to a loss of fluid, sometimes 200–400 mL/hr for someone critically burned. Complicating the sodium shift into the interstitial space, potassium also shifts to this area as it is released from the injured cells. Initially, hyperkalemia is present as fluid resuscitation takes place; however, edema formation decreases and the capillary membrane is no longer permeable. This allows potassium to shift back into the cell. Sodium levels return to normal as fluid shifts back into the vascular space.

NURSING IMPLICATIONS

Assess for signs of decreased tissue perfusion and neurological manifestations of irritability or confusion, indicative of decreased cerebral perfusion. Monitor for cardiac dysrhythmias due to the electrolyte imbalances and fluid shifts that occur. Evaluate laboratory values for hyperkalemia and hyponatremia. The patient may manifest signs of an irregular heart rate, weakness, or diarrhea with hyperkalemia and twitching, seizures, nausea, and vomiting from hyponatremia. Monitor arterial blood gas results assessing for metabolic acidosis. Strict intake and output along with daily weights should be implemented for evaluation of fluid loss.

Intravenous isotonic solutions should be closely monitored for proper fluid replacement. Wound care using strict aseptic technique should follow the protocol of the burn unit.

Decreased tissue perfusion secondary to fluid loss and dehydration are critical events in the burn patient; therefore strict intake and output along with daily weights should be implemented for evaluation of fluid loss. Intravenous isotonic solutions should be closely monitored for proper fluid replacement.

Question: Why is strict aseptic technique important for the burn patient?

Answer: Strict aseptic technique is of utmost importance for the burn patient because the skin barrier, the primary barricade for infection, has been lost.

QUICK LOOK AT THE CHAPTER AHEAD

Shock is a syndrome of life-threatening hemodynamic imbalance leading to poor perfusion and an inadequate supply of oxygen and nutrients to the cells. Different classifications of shock exist, but the pathophysiology for all remains the same. In this chapter we define the different stages of shock and describe the clinical manifestations.

50

Stages of Shock

TERMS
☐ Shock

STAGES OF SHOCK

If detected early on **shock** can be reversed; however, as the shock state progresses the chances of reversing the chain of events become impossible and death ensues. There are three stages of shock (Figure 50-1). The first stage is compensation where changes can be made to reverse the process. Stage II is the progressive stage, indicating that perfusion disturbance has increased and may lead to the third stage, the refractory stage, or a condition that can no longer be reversed.

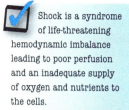

Shock is a syndrome of life-threatening hemodynamic imbalance leading to poor perfusion and an inadequate supply of oxygen and nutrients to the cells.

Stage I: Compensation

As stage I begins the body's metabolic needs are still being met through adequate perfusion, but as the blood pressure decreases compensatory

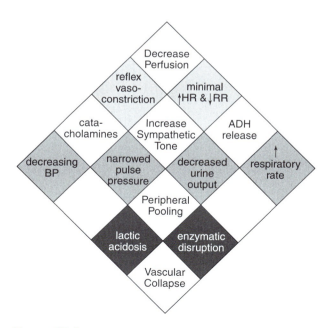

Figure 50-1 Stages of shock.

mechanisms take over. Once the sympathetic nervous system (SNS) is alerted to a decreasing blood pressure, peripheral vasoconstriction maintains blood flow to the major organs, particularly the brain and heart. A mild increase in heart rate helps to increase cardiac output, and dilation of the coronary arteries allows for an increased delivery of oxygen to the cardiac muscle.

 Though compensatory mechanisms take over in the first stage of shock, keeping the major organs perfused comes at a cost to other systems.

Keeping the major organs perfused comes at a cost to other systems. Blood flow to the kidneys is decreased, which activates the release of renin, which activates angiotensinogen to become angiotensin II, a potent vasoconstrictor. Aldosterone is stimulated to increase sodium reabsorption, and the release of antidiuretic hormone increases water resorption. The hormones of the SNS, epinephrine and norepinephrine, also cause vasoconstriction to the blood vessels. All these mechanisms help to increase blood volume to the heart and vital organs, but blood flow to other body systems is diminished.

Capillary hydrostatic pressure becomes decreased and falls below the colloidal osmotic pressure. This allows fluid to flow from the interstitial to the intravascular space, helping to increase blood volume and pressure.

Catecholamines are released to stimulate the liver to release its glycogen stores as the pancreas decreases its release of insulin. This allows an increased amount of glucose for the brain to use for energy during this time.

Question: How does the body attempt to increase blood pressure when shock takes place?

Answer: Angiotensin II and the SNS hormones, potent vasoconstrictors, are activated. Antidiuretic hormone is released to increase water resorption and capillary hydrostatic pressure decreases, allowing fluid to flow into the intravascular space.

Clinical Manifestations of Stage I

During this stage subtle changes occur that can be easily overlooked. The patient is usually oriented to person, time, and place with clear speech but may appear to be somewhat restless and anxious (Table 50-1). Irritability may be present. There may be a subtle drop in blood pressure,

Table 50-1 Clinical Manifestations of Shock

Stage I
  Alert and oriented to person, time, and place
  Restless/anxious/irritable
  Slight ↓ in blood pressure and ↑ in heart rate
  Narrowing pulse pressure
  Urine output normal or slightly ↓
  Acid–base normal

Stage II
  Hypoxia
  Slurred speech
  ↑ Thirst
  Vasoconstriction/cool clammy skin
  ↑ Narrowing of pulse pressure
  ↑ Heart rate/weak thready pulse
  ↓ Cardiac output and blood pressure
  ↓ Urine output
  Anaerobic metabolism = lactic acid
  Acid–base = metabolic acidosis
  ↑ Respiratory rate
  Hyperkalemia
  Possible cardiac dysrhythmias

Stage III
  Unresponsiveness
  Extreme hypotension
  ↑ Vasodilation = blood pooling in periphery
  ↑ Anaerobic metabolism = ↑ lactic acid production
  Metabolic and respiratory acidosis
  Compensatory mechanism nonfunctioning
  Multiple organ dysfunction
  Cardiac output unable to maintain tissue perfusion = cardiac
    and respiratory arrest

↑, Increased; ↓, decreased.

along with an increase in heart rate. A characteristic sign is a narrowing of the pulse pressure, the difference between the systolic and diastolic pressures. The pulse pressure is an indicator of stroke volume, and a narrowed difference between the two pressures indicates a decrease in stroke volume. Urine output may remain normal or may show a

The pulse pressure is the difference between the systolic and diastolic pressures. A narrowed difference between the two pressures indicates a decrease in stroke volume, which indicates a decrease in cardiac output.

slight decrease due to the activation of antidiuretic hormone. Acid–base balance should remain unaffected.

Stage I is the easiest stage to arrest the progression of the shock state. However, it is difficult to recognize stage I because most of the signs are subtle. Many of these signs may not be present, and the patient may easily slide into stage II before one is alerted to the possibility that problems exist.

 Stage I is the easiest stage to arrest the progression of the shock state. However, it is difficult to recognize stage I because most of the signs are subtle.

Stage II: Progressive

The progressive stage occurs when the compensatory mechanisms fail to maintain an adequate cellular perfusion and the initial signs of shock become more pronounced. Vasoconstriction becomes more apparent as the renin-angiotensin mechanism continues to respond to the low blood pressure. Cardiac output and blood pressure further

 The progressive stage occurs when the compensatory mechanisms fail to maintain an adequate cellular perfusion, and the initial signs of shock become more pronounced.

decrease, resulting in tissue hypoxia, which causes anaerobic metabolism and the production of lactic acid. Carbon dioxide cannot be removed due to poor blood flow; consequently, the level of acid in the body rises with the accumulation of intracellular carbonic acid. The kidneys contribute to this worsening situation through impaired renal excretion of H^+. As the level of acidosis increases, electrolytes become imbalanced, particularly potassium, and affect myocardial contractility.

Clinical Manifestations of Stage II
Hypoxia dulls the SNS responses so the patient is oriented to person but becomes easily confused. Speech may be slurred, and the patient may complain of thirst and dry lips and mouth (see Table 50-1). A decreased response to painful stimuli occurs. The skin begins to feel cool and appears pale as vasoconstriction becomes more intense. The systolic blood pressure continues to fall, and the pulse pressure continues to narrow. The heart rate becomes increasingly tachycardic, and the pulse feels weak and thready. Because of all the vasoconstrictive measures, urine output now becomes obviously decreased to approximately 20–30 cc/hr. The respiratory system attempts to decrease the acidosis by increasing respirations to blow off carbon dioxide and lower the carbonic acid level.

Stage III: Refractory

The third stage of shock is virtually irreversible. The patient is unresponsive and compensatory mechanisms are no longer functioning, the blood pressure cannot be maintained, and

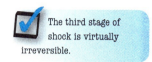

The third stage of shock is virtually irreversible.

a syndrome of multiple organ dysfunction occurs. Every system is compromised and becomes dysfunctional. Even if the cells were able to receive oxygen the mitochondria of the cell is now so severely damaged that the cell is unable to use the oxygen. The cascade of effects is overwhelming, and the body is unable to recover.

Clinical Manifestations of Stage III

An anaerobic metabolism occurs secondary to a lack of oxygen, which contributes to the production of lactic acid and a metabolic/respiratory acidotic state (see Table 50-1). The SNS can no longer maintain its measures for vasoconstriction, and a loss of sympathetic tone allows blood to pool in the periphery. Blood also pools in the capillaries, creating a movement of fluid out of the vascular space that furthers the hypotension. Cardiac output becomes too low to maintain cerebral, cardiac, respiratory, and renal perfusion. Underperfused and needing oxygen, the tissues suffer from the insult of a severe acidosis and cellular ischemia and death, leading to cardiac and respiratory arrest.

QUICK LOOK AT THE CHAPTER AHEAD

Shock is generally classified into three categories, cardiogenic, circulatory, and distributive. In this chapter we look at these three different types of shock along with the fluid, electrolyte, and acid–base imbalances and nursing implications of all shock states.

51

Types of Shock

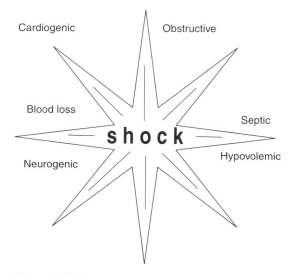

Figure 51-1 Shock.

CATEGORIES OF SHOCK

Shock is generally classified into three categories (Table 51-1). **Cardiogenic shock** is the inability of the heart to pump blood throughout the body. **Circulatory shock** is the loss of intravascular volume and has two subclassifications, hypovolemic and obstructive. The third main classification is distributive shock, which includes subclassifications of neurogenic, anaphylactic, and septic shock. Regardless of the type of shock, the stages the patient goes through remain the same. The compensatory mechanisms do not change because the outcome for all types, if uncorrected, is a decreased perfusion resulting in a lack of cellular oxygenation, multiple organ dysfunction, and death.

> ✔ Regardless of the type of shock, the stages the patient goes through remain the same. The compensatory mechanisms do not change because the outcome for all types, if uncorrected, is a decreased perfusion resulting in a lack of cellular oxygenation, multiple organ dysfunction, and death.

Table 51-1 Categories of Shock

Cardiogenic shock = inability of heart to pump blood throughout the body

Circulatory shock = loss of intravascular volume
    Hypovolemic
    Obstructive

Distributive shock = loss of blood vessel tone
    Neurogenic
    Anaphylactic
    Septic

Cardiogenic Shock

Cardiogenic shock is most commonly caused by myocardial infarction. The development of shock depends on the amount of muscle wall damage that results from this insult. Other types of shock causing an inadequate circulation of blood may also lead to cardiogenic shock. When other types of shock

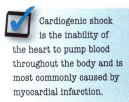

Cardiogenic shock is the inability of the heart to pump blood throughout the body and is most commonly caused by myocardial infarction.

are responsible, a myocardial depressant factor is released that causes a severe depression of the heart's muscle ability to contract, resulting in a dilation of the left ventricle and leading to an inability for the heart to eject a sufficient amount of blood into the circulation.

Treatment

An intraaortic balloon pump is most likely needed to assist the heart in propelling blood through the aorta. Fluid volume walks a tight rope between too much and too little. Hemodynamic monitoring is essential to regulate the intravenous fluids given to the patient. Enough fluid must be administered to keep the preload (ventricular filling pressure) sufficient and yet not too much to overburden an already taxed system. Correction of dysrhythmias and the use of inotropic agents (e.g., dopamine) may be necessary for maintaining blood pressure; however, decreasing the workload of the heart by decreasing afterload (systemic vascular resistance) through vasodilators (e.g., nitroglycerin) is also important.

Circulatory Shock

A loss of circulating blood volume, whether actual or shifted among the fluid compartments, is the cause of circulatory shock. The result is a lack of cellular oxygenation and eventual tissue and organ failure. Two types of circulatory shock are hypovolemic shock and obstructive shock.

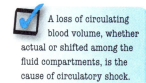

A loss of circulating blood volume, whether actual or shifted among the fluid compartments, is the cause of circulatory shock.

Hypovolemic Shock

Hypovolemic shock occurs when approximately 15–20% of the blood volume is lost. It may occur with trauma in which hemorrhaging and a loss of whole blood occurs, with burns and a loss of plasma, or with a loss of extracellular fluid such as with the gastrointestinal system fluid loss through excessive vomiting or diarrhea. Third spacing, the shifting of fluid from the vascular compartment to the interstitial or intracellular, or internal hemorrhaging also may cause hypovolemic shock.

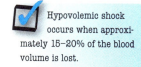

Hypovolemic shock occurs when approximately 15–20% of the blood volume is lost.

Inadequate perfusion, the ultimate outcome of hypovolemic shock, starts with a decreased blood return to the heart and results in a decreased cardiac output and circulatory insufficiency. The compensatory mechanisms of sympathetic nervous system (SNS) stimulation, renin-angiotensin activation, and antidiuretic hormone stimulation attempt to maintain the blood pressure and cardiac output.

Treatment involves rapid fluid replacement. Surgical intervention may be needed if the insult is related to trauma. Success is achieved when blood pressure and cardiac output return to normal. A urine output of approximately 30 cc/hr indicates fluid balance has been achieved.

Obstructive Shock

Obstructive shock is related to some type of mechanical obstruction that interrupts blood flow through the circulation, heart, or lungs. Situations involving dissecting aortic aneurysm, cardiac tamponade, or pulmonary embolism are some of the more common factors causing obstructive shock. The

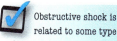

Obstructive shock is related to some type of mechanical obstruction that interrupts blood flow through the circulation, heart, or lungs.

obstruction of blood flow causes the pressures of the right side of the heart to elevate and impairs the return of blood to the heart, resulting in jugular vein distention and an elevated central venous pressure.

Treatment includes correcting the problem and returning blood flow to normal. Maintaining blood pressure and cardiac output during this type of shock is difficult because blood flow is obstructed. Thrombolytics may work with pulmonary embolism, although multiple contraindications such as age, cardiopulmonary resuscitation, and recent surgery may prevent use of this therapy. Surgical repair of an aneurysm or removing fluid from the pericardial sac with tamponade may help to alleviate the blockage.

Distributive Shock

Distributive shock occurs because of an increased vascular compartment related to loss of blood vessel tone. The blood volume then becomes redistributed, and a decreased volume is returned to the heart. This accounts for a decreased cardiac output

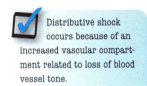

Distributive shock occurs because of an increased vascular compartment related to loss of blood vessel tone.

and blood pressure. The important point to remember in distributive shock is that the blood volume is not diminished but redistributed. Three types of distributive shock exist: neurogenic shock, anaphylactic shock, and septic shock.

Neurogenic Shock

Neurogenic shock occurs secondary to a loss of vasomotor tone that brings about vasodilation. Neurogenic shock may be caused by brain or spinal cord injury from a diving accident or a bullet wound, lack of glucose

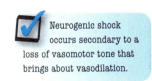

Neurogenic shock occurs secondary to a loss of vasomotor tone that brings about vasodilation.

to the brain, overdose of drugs, or anesthesia. In neurogenic shock the skin is warm and dry. Cervical spinal cord injuries, at or above the fifth thoracic vertebra, result in the loss of SNS vasoconstrictor tone, causing an uncompensated massive vasodilation. In addition, hypotension occurs because of an unopposed parasympathetic nervous system action, allowing for bradycardia, unlike other shock states where tachycardia is a compensatory mechanism. Often, the patient with spinal injury has hypothalamic dysfunction that causes a temperature dysfunction called

poikilothermia (temperature of the environment); when combined with the vasodilation, the patient's temperature becomes even cooler.

Neurogenic shock is rare, and if the cause is known the condition may be corrected; for example, neurogenic shock related to anesthesia can be reversed. Temporary administration of vasoconstrictors such as dopamine may be indicated. An insulin reaction causing decreased glucose availability for the brain can also be easily reversed through administration of glucose. Spinal cord injury is permanent, and treatment of the shock state is comprehensive. Neurogenic shock related to spinal cord injury can develop immediately after the injury and last for days to weeks. Treatment involves fluid resuscitation and vasopressors such as dopamine to maintain cardiac output and tissue perfusion, phenylephrine or norepinephrine to increase the systemic vascular resistance, and management of the hypothermia with heating blankets.

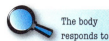

The body responds to most shock states through vasoconstriction to help pull blood volume to the vital organs, thus leaving the skin cool and clammy. In neurogenic shock, secondary to spinal injuries at or above the fifth thoracic vertebra, the skin is warm and dry due to the loss of SNS, resulting in massive vasodilation.

Anaphylactic Shock

Anaphylactic shock occurs when vasodilators such as histamine are released into the circulation as a result of an allergic reaction to drugs, foods, insect stings, or antitoxins. The release of vasoactive mediators causes the vasodilation of arterioles and venules and makes the capillary wall permeable, which results in the leaking of fluid from the vascular to the interstitial space.

Anaphylaxis occurs when vasodilators such as histamine are released into the circulation as a result of an allergic reaction to drugs, foods, insect stings, or antitoxins.

Initially, respiratory problems such as coughing, wheezing, and difficulty breathing occur. Bronchospasm and laryngeal edema develop, causing serious airway obstruction. Depending on the cause, itching and swelling of the lips, tongue, and eyes may occur. As with all distributive shock the blood vessels dilate and the blood pools in the periphery, causing a decreased blood pressure and cardiac output.

Treatment includes prompt intervention with maintaining an open airway and oxygenation. Removing the cause is difficult because the insect bite or ingestion of substance has already occurred. Epinephrine or other antihistamines are essential for constricting blood vessels, smooth muscle relaxation to assist bronchodilation, and blockage of histamines.

Septic Shock

Septic shock is one of the most prevalent types of shock affecting hospitalized patients, though it can occur with healthy individuals who contract microorganisms that enter the bloodstream. As one of the most common types of distributive shock, it has a mortality rate of 50%. Hospitalized patients are most susceptible due to the use of invasive technology allowing for a portal of entry for the microorganism, coupled with an already immunocompromised system. The elderly are particularly susceptible because of a compromised immune system secondary to age and chronic diseases. Patients undergoing chemotherapy whose immune systems become compromised from the drugs are vulnerable to microorganisms and potential sepsis.

Septic shock stems from an infection caused primarily by gram-negative bacteria; however, gram-positive bacteria such as *Staphylococcus aureus,* which are usually responsible for toxic shock, can also be the cause of septic shock. Regardless of the type of bacteria, the microorganism triggers components that release a cascade of events. Several theories exist that attempt to explain the body's reaction to the microorganism. One theory speaks to toxins released from the microorganism that cause an immune reaction responsible for decreased vascular tone and increased permeability of the vascular system. This allows for a decreased systemic vascular resistance and vasodilation that contributes to a maldistribution of the circulating blood volume and the hypotension that accompanies shock states. Another theory refers to systems such as complement, kinin, and the clotting cascade that, once released, cause widespread complications such as an increased permeability of the capillary wall and the development of the clotting syndrome, disseminated intravascular coagulation.

 Septic shock stems from an infection caused primarily by gram-negative bacteria; however, gram-positive bacteria such as Staphylococcus aureus, which are usually responsible for toxic shock, can also be the cause of septic shock.

The clinical presentation of septic shock varies somewhat from the other types of shock. In the initial stages of septic shock the patient looks uncompromised and may appear this way for hours to days before the start of the next stage. The skin is warm and dry with a rosy appearance due to the start of a decreased systemic vascular resistance and vasodilation. Personality changes and irritability may be present due to decreased cerebral blood flow. Respiratory alkalosis may also be present due to a slight hyperventilation. Urine output may be up to 100 cc/hr. Typically, the patient has a fever. The presentation of the patient in the initial stages of septic shock is that of a hyperdynamic state with a higher than normal cardiac output (compensatory mechanism for the decreased systemic vascular resistance) and normal to slightly decreased blood pressure and increased heart rate. However, if the shock progresses, increased vasodilation contributes to a lower blood pressure and the heart becomes dilated, unable to eject the necessary amount of blood required for adequate tissue perfusion.

 The clinical presentation of septic shock is somewhat different from the other types of shock in that a hyperdynamic state occurs, making the skin warm and dry, taking on a rosy appearance. This may be deceiving, making the patient look healthy when he or she is actually in the initial stage of septic shock.

 A good clue to being alert to the initial stage of shock is a change in the patient's personality such as irritability, confusion, or restlessness.

Treatment consists of identification of the source of infection and administration of broad-spectrum and aminoglycoside antibiotics. Rapid infusion of intravenous fluids and vasopressor drugs to help increase the systemic vascular resistance is of importance. Hemodynamic monitoring to monitor fluid balance is absolutely essential.

FLUID, ELECTROLYTE, AND ACID-BASE IMBALANCES IN SHOCK STATES

The fluid and electrolyte imbalances that occur with shock are vast. The blood urea nitrogen and creatinine elevate because of hypoperfusion and vasoconstriction of the renal system. Sodium increases during the early stages secondary to the increased secretion of aldosterone, but potassium decreases with renal excretion. Potassium increases as shock progresses because of the exchange with hydrogen ions in acidosis and the release of potassium with cellular death. Calcium also increases in an acidotic state.

Acid–base balance swings from an alkalotic state to one of acidosis as the stages of shock progress. A respiratory alkalosis occurs during the beginning stages because of hyperventilation. Metabolic acidosis quickly ensues, however, with the accumulation of lactic acid from anaerobic metabolism.

NURSING IMPLICATIONS

As mentioned throughout this chapter, different types of shock states involve varied medical treatment. Regardless of the type of shock, however, there are basic nursing assessments and interventions that are appropriate.

Neurological checks and evaluation of the patient's level of consciousness are important indicators of cerebral blood flow. Behavioral manifestations of restlessness, irritability, confusion, and paresthesias are indicators of decreased cerebral blood flow. In addition to performing a neurological assessment every hour, recording and reporting abnormal deviations and protecting the patient from injury are essential interventions.

Airway is of primary importance, particularly with anaphylactic shock but also with other shock-like states. Assessment of an increased and/or decreased rate, shallow and/or increased depth, use of accessory muscles or adventitious breath sounds, cyanosis, or dyspnea are indicators of respiratory distress. Administration of oxygen and ventilatory assistance may be required. Pulse oximetry to evaluate oxygen saturation and arterial blood gases for acid–base balance should be monitored. The lactic acidosis that develops with shock states does not require treatment with sodium bicarbonate unless the pH falls below 7.2. Generally, supplementary oxygen helps to increase tissue perfusion, and fluid replacement helps to correct the acidotic state.

Assessment of vital signs, pulmonary artery pressures, pulmonary artery wedge pressures, and cardiac output are necessary, every 15 minutes if needed (pulmonary artery wedge pressure is not taken as frequently due to complications with balloon rupture) and every hour as the patient stabilizes. Low blood pressure, postural hypotension, tachycardia or weak thready pulse, low pulmonary artery pressures, and decreased urinary output are all indicators of fluid imbalance. Inotropic agents such as dopamine need to be titrated to support blood pressure. Cardiac monitoring is essential to prevent lethal dysrhythmias from developing secondary to electrolyte, acid–base, and fluid imbalances.

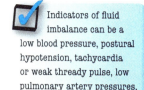

Indicators of fluid imbalance can be a low blood pressure, postural hypotension, tachycardia or weak thready pulse, low pulmonary artery pressures, or decreased urinary output.

With the exception of cardiogenic shock, fluids such as normal saline are essential for volume expansion. Increased amounts of crystalloids are required because much of the volume diffuses out of the vascular space secondary to increased capillary permeability and decreased oncotic pressure. Crystalloids, as large molecules, are unable to leave the intravascular space and, in addition, attract fluid, helping to expand the intravascular compartment. Intake and output should be carefully measured on an hourly basis.

Question: Why are crystalloids helpful for volume expansion?

Answer: Crystalloids, as large molecules, are unable to leave the intravascular space and, in addition, attract fluid, helping to expand the intravascular compartment.

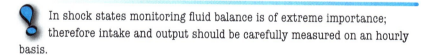

In shock states monitoring fluid balance is of extreme importance; therefore intake and output should be carefully measured on an hourly basis.

Monitoring signs and symptoms of overload through pulmonary artery/wedge pressures and urine output is important for evaluating renal function and to help assess fluid balance and adequate replacement. Measure urine output every hour. Assess and report laboratory values of elevated serum blood urea nitrogen and creatinine, low urine sodium, or blood in urine, all indicators of inadequate renal function.

Assessing for the presence of bowel sounds, distension, or abdominal pain should be conducted every 4 hours. Report problems of nausea and vomiting or diarrhea, all potential contributors to acid–base and electrolyte imbalances. Enteral feedings should be started as soon as the patient can tolerate to meet metabolic demands.

Assess for peripheral vascular ischemia. Palpate all peripheral pulses and document and report complaints of pain, tingling, or numbness in the extremities. Evaluate the skin for pale or cyanotic color and for temperature as well as dryness. Helping the patient maintain a normal temperature provides comfort and prevents vasoconstriction. Proper skin care to maintain skin integrity is also important when the patient is immobile.

Fear and anxiety are concerns of the patient when aware of the severity of the situation. Assessing for sleeplessness, lack of communication, restlessness, or an increase in vital signs may indicate anxiety or a fear of death. Acknowledging the patient's feelings and showing concern help to calm the patient and reduce anxiety.

PART V · QUESTIONS

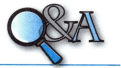

1. The most common cause of acute renal failure is
   (A) Hypertension
   (B) Nephrotoxic injury
   (C) Calculi
   (D) Acute tubular necrosis

2. An example of a prerenal factor that may cause acute renal failure is
   (A) Clamping the aorta for more than 30 minutes during surgery
   (B) Radiocontrast dyes
   (C) Prostatic hyperplasia
   (D) Renal tumor

3. Hyperkalemia in chronic renal failure results from _____ and _____.
   (A) Oliguria, acidosis
   (B) Increased urine output, low calcium levels
   (C) Increased phosphate levels, low calcium levels
   (D) Increased urine output, increased magnesium levels

4. Low levels of calcium occur in chronic renal failure due to
   (A) A decreased production of erythropoietin
   (B) Elevated levels of phosphate
   (C) Lack of vitamin D normally created by the kidneys
   (D) An osmotic diuresis related to sodium loss

5. A V/Q mismatch is
   (A) An anatomical shunt
   (B) A ventilation-perfusion discrepancy
   (C) Decreased oxygen levels and increased alveolar carbon dioxide levels
   (D) An inability to expel carbon dioxide

6. Which of the following is a sign of right-sided heart failure?
   (A) Blood backing up into the pulmonary bed
   (B) Elevated pulmonary artery wedge pressure
   (C) Jugular venous distension and peripheral edema
   (D) Decreased urine output

7. One of the hallmark signs of diabetic ketoacidosis is
   (A) Hypertension
   (B) Too much insulin
   (C) Too few ketones
   (D) Fruity breath

8. Dehydration from HHNK syndrome results from
   (A) Lack of insulin
   (B) Elevated glucose levels
   (C) Excess ketones
   (D) Acidosis

9. Which of the following would indicate a deep partial-thickness burn injury?
   (A) Mottled waxy appearance
   (B) Red, shiny, wet appearance
   (C) Charred and dry
   (D) Erythema and intact skin

10. Which stage of shock is the easiest stage to reverse the chain of events that lead to serious complications?
    (A) Progressive
    (B) Refractory
    (C) Compensation
    (D) Syndrome of multiple organ dysfunction

11. Which of the following types of shock is a redistribution of blood, not a loss of volume?
    (A) Hypovolemic shock
    (B) Distributive shock
    (C) Cardiogenic shock
    (D) Obstructive shock

12. The patient has a rosy appearance and the skin is warm and dry during the beginning phases of septic shock due to
    (A) Vasoconstriction
    (B) Hypertension
    (C) Increased vascular tone
    (D) Vasodilation

PART V • ANSWERS AND RATIONALES

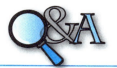

1. The correct answer is D.
Rationale: The most common cause of acute renal failure is acute tubular necrosis. Calculi, injury caused by medications, and hypertension do take their toll on the kidney.

2. The correct answer is A.
Rationale: A prerenal cause for acute renal failure takes place outside of the renal system, causing a decreased blood flow to the kidneys. If blood flow is restored in time, damage to the kidneys is minimal. Radiocontrast dyes are an example of an intrarenal factor causing damage to the renal tissue/nephrons of the kidneys. Prostatic hyperplasia and renal tumor are examples of postrenal factors that cause an obstruction to the urological structures.

3. The correct answer is A.
Rationale: Potassium is eliminated in the urine, and when little urine output exists potassium accumulates. Also, during acidosis the hydrogen ion moves into the cell in exchange for the potassium ion, contributing to the state of hyperkalemia. An increased urine output does not exist in chronic renal failure, and the levels of calcium, magnesium, and phosphate are affected but do not contribute to hyperkalemia.

4. The correct answer is C.
Rationale: The kidneys need to activate vitamin D for the gastrointestinal system to absorb calcium. Because the kidneys lose that function in chronic renal failure, calcium is not absorbed and hypocalcemia results. The low calcium triggers the release of parathyroid hormone, which also releases phosphate, contributing to the high phosphate levels. Erythropoietin is a hormone produced by the kidneys that affects the red blood cell. Low calcium levels are not related to an osmotic diuresis.

5. The correct answer is B.
Rationale: Ventilation and perfusion should be close to a 1:1 ratio. In certain respiratory conditions ventilation may be affected and in others perfusion may be blocked, leading to a V/Q mismatch.

An anatomical shunt occurs when blood enters the left side of the heart without passing through the lungs. Decreased oxygen levels and increased alveolar carbon dioxide refer to alveolar hypoventilation. An inability to expel carbon dioxide refers to hypercapnic respiratory failure.

6. The correct answer is C.

Rationale: Peripheral edema and jugular venous distension are signs of blood backing up in the peripheral or systemic circulation from a failing right ventricle. Answers A and B are related to left-sided failure, though eventually they can be the cause of right-sided failure. A decreased urine output is not a sign of congestive heart failure; it may be associated with another disease process such as chronic renal failure in conjunction with congestive heart failure.

7. The correct answer is D.

Rationale: The fruity breath is related to the excess ketones in the body, and the breath takes on the smell of apple seeds (acetone). The condition results from too little insulin in relation to increased caloric intake or stress. Hypotension is common, not hypertension. Hypotension develops along with a weak rapid pulse due to low volume secondary to an increased urine output.

8. The correct answer is B.

Rationale: The elevated glucose causes an osmotic diuresis that leads to dehydration. The condition occurs with patients who are capable of producing insulin, but not enough to counteract excess glucose. The main difference between DKA and HHNK syndrome is the lack of ketones and acidosis as is present with HHNK syndrome.

9. The correct answer is A.

Rationale: The second-degree deep partial-thickness injury takes on a mottled waxy-white or pink color with thin paper-like blisters. Answer B is a second-degree superficial partial-thickness burn. These injuries have skin that appears moist and weepy with blisters. Answer C is a fourth-degree burn, and answer D is a first-degree burn.

10. The correct answer is C.

Rationale: The compensatory stage is the initial stage when the body's compensatory mechanisms are attempting to keep up with the evolving process. Interceding at this stage is easiest because changes in vital signs, urine output, and so on are still subtle. The progressive stage begins to show a decrease in cardiac output, blood pressure, and an accumulation of acid. The refractory stage is virtually irreversible.

11. The correct answer is B.

Rationale: Distributive shock occurs because the vascular compartment size has increased through lost vessel tone, redistributing the blood volume. Hypovolemic shock is an actual loss of blood volume. Cardiogenic shock is related to the inability of the heart to effectively pump blood to the tissues. Obstructive shock is related to a mechanical obstruction interrupting blood flow.

12. The correct answer is D.

Rationale: The skin is warm and dry with a rosy appearance due to vasodilation. The vasodilation occurs due to a decreased vascular tone, allowing for more blood to pool into the peripheral areas and away from the major organs. Vasoconstriction leads to cool clammy skin because the blood is shunted away from the periphery. Hypertension does not occur in shock.

References and
Glossary

REFERENCES

Part I

Corwin, E.J. (2008). *Handbook of pathophysiology* (3rd ed.). Philadelphia: Lippincott.

Hogan, M.A. (ed.). (2007). *Fluids, electrolytes, & acid-base balance* (2nd ed.). New Jersey: Prentice Hall.

Kaplan, J. (2002). Biochemistry of Na, K-ATPase. *Annual Review of Biochemistry, 71*, 511–535.

Lewis, S., Heitkemper, M., Dirksen, S., O'Brien, P., Giddens, J., & Bucher, L. (2004). *Medical-surgical nursing assessment and management of clinical problems* (6th ed.). St. Louis: Mosby.

McCance, K., & Huether, S. (2006). *Pathophysiology: The biologic basis for disease in adults and children* (5th ed.). Mosby: St. Louis.

Porth, C. (2004). *Pathophysiology concepts of altered health states* (7th ed.). Philadelphia: Lippincott.

Price, S., & Wilson, L. (2003). *Pathophysiology clinical concepts of disease processes* (6th ed). St. Louis: Mosby.

Part II

American Heart Association. Retrieved 8/30/06 from http://www.americanheart.org

Beck, L. (2000). The aging kidney: Defending a delicate balance of fluid and electrolytes. *Geriatrics, 55*(4), 26–32.

Bigard, A.X., Sanchez, H., & Claveyrolas, G. (2001). Effects of dehydration and rehydration on EMG changes during fatiguing contractions. *Medicine and Science in Sports and Exercise, 33*(10), 1694–1700.

Carroll, M., & Schade, D. (2003). A practical approach to hypercalcemia. *American Family Physician, 67,* 1959–1966.

Castiglione, V. (2000). Emergency hyperkalemia. *American Journal of Nursing, 100*(1), 55–56.

Corwin, E.J. (2008). *Handbook of pathophysiology* (3rd ed.). Philadelphia: Lippincott.

Gisolfi, C., Lambert, P., & Summers, R. (2001). Intestinal fluid absorption during exercise: Role of sport drink osmolality and (Na$^+$). *Medicine and Science in Sports and Exercise, 33*(6), 907–915.

Hogan, M.A. (ed.). (2007). *Fluids, electrolytes, & acid-base balance* (2nd ed.). New Jersey: Prentice Hall.

Kaplow, R., & Hardin, S.R. (2007). *Critical care nursing synergy for optimal outcomes.* Sudbury, MA: Jones and Bartlett.

Lewis, S., Heitkemper, M., Dirkesen, S., O'Brien, P., Giddens, J., & Bucher, L. (2004). *Medical-surgical nursing assessment and management of clinical problems* (6th ed.). St. Louis: Mosby.

Mao, I.F., Chen, M.-L., & Ko, Y.C. (2001). Electrolyte loss in sweat and iodine deficiency in a hot environment. *Archives of Environmental Health, 56*(3), 271–277.

McCance, K., & Huether, S. (2006). *Pathophysiology: The biologic basis for disease in adults and children* (5th ed.). St. Louis: Mosby.

Messinger-Rapport, B., & Thacker, H. (2002). Prevention for older women: A practical guide to prevention and treatment of osteoporosis. *Geriatrics, 57*(4), 16–27.

Porth, C. (2004). *Pathophysiology concepts of altered health states* (7th ed.). Philadelphia: Lippincott.

Price, S., & Wilson, L. (2003). *Pathophysiology clinical concepts of disease processes* (6th ed). St. Louis: Mosby.

Stephanides, S.L. (2005 December 14). *Hypernatremia.* Retrieved December 14, 2006 from http://eMedicine.

The minerals we need. (2003). *Harvard Women's Health Watch, 10*(9), 5–6.

Urden, L.D., Stacy, K.M., & Lough, M.E. (2006). *Thelan's critical care nursing* (5th ed.). St. Louis: Mosby.

U.S. Department of Agriculture, Agricultural Research Service. (2003). USDA national nutrient database for standard reference, release 16. Nutrient data laboratory home page, http://www.ars.usda.gov/ba/bhnrc/ndl

Wexler, R. (2002). Evaluation and treatment of heat-related illnesses. *American Family Physician, 65*(11), 2307–2314.

Part III

Corwin, E.J. (2008). *Handbook of pathophysiology* (3rd ed.). Philadelphia: Lippincott.

Hogan, M.A. (ed.). (2007). *Fluids, electrolytes, & acid-base balance* (2nd ed.). New Jersey: Prentice Hall.

Kaplan, J. (2002). Biochemistry of Na, K-ATPase. *Annual Review of Biochemistry, 71*, 511–535.

Lewis, S., Heitkemper, M., Dirkesen, S., O'Brien, P., Giddens, J., & Bucher, L. (2004). *Medical-surgical nursing assessment and management of clinical problems* (6th ed.). St. Louis: Mosby.

McCance, K., & Huether, S. (2006). *Pathophysiology: The biologic basis for disease in adults and children* (5th ed.). St. Louis: Mosby.

Porth, C. (2004). *Pathophysiology concepts of altered health states* (7th ed.). Philadelphia: Lippincott.

Price, S., & Wilson, L. (2003). *Pathophysiology clinical concepts of disease processes* (6th ed). St. Louis: Mosby.

Stephens, T., McKenna, M., & Canny, B. (2002). Effect of sodium bicarbonate on muscle metabolism during intense endurance cycling. *Medicine and Science in Sports and Exercise, 34*(4), 614–621.

Urden, L.D., Stacy, K.M., & Lough, M.E. (2006). *Thelan's critical care nursing* (5th ed.). St. Louis: Mosby.

Part IV

Corwin, E.J. (2008). *Handbook of pathophysiology* (3rd ed.). Philadelphia: Lippincott.

Hogan, M.A. (ed.). (2007). *Fluids, electrolytes, & acid-base balance* (2nd ed.). New Jersey: Prentice Hall.

Kaplan, J. (2002). Biochemistry of Na, K-ATPase. *Annual Review of Biochemistry, 71,* 511–535.

Kaplow, R., & Hardin, S.R. (2007). *Critical care nursing synergy for optimal outcomes.* Sudbury, MA: Jones and Bartlett.

Lewis, S., Heitkemper, M., Dirkesen, S., O'Brien, P., Giddens, J., & Bucher, L. (2004). *Medical-surgical nursing assessment and management of clinical problems* (6th ed.). St. Louis: Mosby.

McCance, K., & Huether, S. (2006). *Pathophysiology: The biologic basis for disease in adults and children* (5th ed.). St. Louis: Mosby.

Newberry, L. (ed.). (2003). *Sheehy's emergency nursing: Principles and practice* (5th ed.). St Louis: Mosby-Yearbook.

Porth, C. (2004). *Pathophysiology concepts of altered health states* (7th ed.). Philadelphia: Lippincott.

Price, S., & Wilson, L. (2003). *Pathophysiology clinical concepts of disease processes* (6th ed.). St. Louis: Mosby.

Urden, L.D., Stacy, K.M., & Lough, M.E. (2006). *Thelan's critical care nursing* (5th ed.). St. Louis: Mosby.

Part V

Ammon, S. (2001). Managing patients with heart failure. *American Journal of Nursing, 101*(12), 26–33.

Beck, L. (2000). The aging kidney: Defending a delicate balance of fluid and electrolytes. *Geriatrics, 55*(4), 26–32.

Broscious, S.K., & Castagnola, J.C. (2006). Chronic kidney disease: Acute manifestations and role of critical care nurses. *Critical Care Nurse, 26*(4), 17–28.

Carelock, J., & Clark, A. (2001). Heart failure: Pathophysiologic mechanisms. *American Journal of Nursing, 101*(12), 26–33.

Corwin, E.J. (2008). *Handbook of pathophysiology* (3rd ed.). Philadelphia: Lippincott.

Dinwiddle, L.C., Burrows-Hudson, S., & Peacock, E.J. (2006). Stage 4 chronic kidney disease. *American Journal of Nursing, 106*(9), 40–51.

Futterman, L., & Lemberg, L. (2003). Diuretics, the most critical therapy in heart failure, yet often neglected in the literature. *American Journal of Critical Care, 121*(4), 376–380.

Hogan, M.A. (ed.). (2007). *Fluids, electrolytes, & acid-base balance* (2nd ed.). New Jersey: Prentice Hall.

Kaplan, J. (2002). Biochemistry of Na, K-ATPase. *Annual Review of Biochemistry, 71*, 511–535.

Kaplow, R., & Hardin, S.R. (2007). *Critical care nursing synergy for optimal outcomes.* Sudbury, MA: Jones and Bartlett.

Lee, C.S. (2006). Role of exogenous arginine vasopressin in the management of catecholamine-refractory septic shock. *Critical Care Nurse, 26*(6), 17–23.

Lewis, S., Heitkemper, M., Dirkesen, S., O'Brien, P., Giddens, J., & Bucher, L. (2004). *Medical-surgical nursing assessment and management of clinical problems* (6th ed.). St. Louis: Mosby.

Marks, J.B. (2003). Perioperative management of diabetes. *American Family Physician, 67*(1), 93–100.

McCance, K., & Huether, S. (2006). *Pathophysiology: The biologic basis for disease in adults and children* (5th ed.). St. Louis: Mosby.

Newberry, L. (ed.). (2003). *Sheehy's emergency nursing: Principles and practice* (5th ed.). St. Louis: Mosby-Yearbook.

Picard, K.M., O'Donoghue, S.C., Young-Kershaw, D.A., & Russell, K.J. (2006). Development and implementation of a multidisciplinary sepsis protocol. *Critical Care Nurse, 26*(3), 43–54.

Porth, C. (2004). *Pathophysiology concepts of altered health states* (7th ed.). Philadelphia: Lippincott.

Price, S., & Wilson, L. (2003). *Pathophysiology clinical concepts of disease processes* (6th ed.). St. Louis: Mosby.

Stefanidis, I., Stiller, S., Ikonomov, V., & Mann, H. (2002). Sodium and body fluid homeostasis in profiling hemodialysis treatment. *The International Journal of Artificial Organs, 25*(5), 421–428.

Urden, L.D., Stacy, K.M., & Lough, M.E. (2006). *Thelan's critical care nursing* (5th ed.). St. Louis: Mosby.

GLOSSARY

Acid: A substance that acts as a donor of a hydrogen ion.

Active transport: The use of energy to move molecules.

Acute renal failure: Related to a sudden decrease in the glomerular filtration rate causing a low urine output.

Adenosine triphosphate: A primary source of energy for moving compounds in and out of the cells.

Aldosterone: A mineralocorticoid secreted when blood volume is low to help regulate sodium balance.

Anaphylactic shock: A shock state that occurs when vasodilators are released into the circulation as a result of an allergic reaction.

Anasarca: Dependent edema beginning in the sacrum and lower extremities and becoming generalized throughout the body.

Anion: Negatively charged ion.

Antidiuretic hormone: A hormone secreted by the posterior pituitary gland in response to stimulation from the hypothalamus secondary to increased fluid osmolality.

Atrial natriuretic peptide: Hormone released when the atria of the heart muscle are overly stretched due to fluid overload.

Base: A substance that consists of molecules that accept the hydrogen ion.

Calcium: HA mineral that helps to build and maintain the bones and teeth, regulate the heart's rhythm, transmit nerve impulses, and assist with blood clotting.

Capillary hydrostatic pressure: Vascular fluid pushing solutes and fluids through a capillary wall produced by the pumping action of the heart.

Cardiogenic shock: Inability of the heart to pump blood through the body. Most commonly caused by myocardial infarction.

Cation: Positively charged ion.

Cell: The smallest autonomous functional unit of the body.

Cell coat: Glycoproteins, glycolipids, and lectins that form the outside surface of the cell that help in cell-to-cell recognition and adhesion.

Cell membrane: A semipermeable membrane that separates the intracellular from the extracellular components, allowing for an exchange of materials through the membrane.

Chloride: A mineral electrolyte found primarily in the extracellular fluid that helps distribute body fluids by joining with sodium and water.

Chloride shift: The movement of chloride into the cell to provide a negative charge for electrical neutrality when large amounts of bicarbonate are drawn into the plasma to act as a buffering mechanism.

Chronic renal failure: Irreversible destruction of the nephrons of both kidneys.

Chvostek's sign: Twitching of the upper lip, nose, eye, and facial muscles when the facial nerve is tapped approximately 2 cm anterior to the tragus of the ear.

Circulatory shock: The loss of intravascular volume. Circulatory shock may be subclassified as hypovolemic or obstructive.

Colloidal osmotic (oncotic) pressure: The force supplied by high-molecular-weight serum proteins, such as albumin, that are too large to escape through the capillary walls.

Concentration gradient: The difference in concentration between an area of greater solute concentration and an area of lesser solute concentration.

Cor pulmonale: Right ventricular enlargement secondary to lung disease.

Diabetes insipidus: An inability to concentrate urine resulting in a state of polyuria. Causes of diabetes insipidus may be neurogenic or nephrogenic.

Diabetes mellitus: A group of heterogeneous disorders that affect carbohydrate metabolism and glucose homeostasis.

Diabetic ketoacidosis: A serious complication of diabetes mellitus where the patient manifests a blood glucose > 250 mg/dL, serum pH < 7.3, serum HCO_3 < 15 mEq/L, and ketonemia or ketonuria.

Diastolic failure: When the ventricles become unable to sufficiently relax and fill completely, resulting in a decreased amount of oxygenated blood returning from the lungs to the heart.

Diffusion: The movement of solutes from a state of higher concentration to that of a lower concentration.

Distributive shock: A shock state that occurs secondary to an increased vascular compartment related to a loss of blood vessel tone.

Dyspnea: Difficulty breathing.

Edema: Common term associated with fluid overload found in the interstitial or lung tissue.

Extracellular fluid: Fluid outside the cell that is divided into the interstitial and the intravascular compartments.

First-degree burn: Burn injury that destroys the outer layer of the epidermis but the skin remains intact.

Fourth-degree burn: Burn injury destroying all layers of the skin including muscle and bone.

Glomerular filtration: The filtering of fluids and solutes through the glomerulus of the kidney.

Heart failure: An abnormal condition of the heart's ability to pump blood to meet the metabolic needs of the tissues.

Hydrogen ion: Needed for maintenance of cellular membranes and enzyme reactions (acid).

Hypercalcemia: Results when the movement of calcium into the circulation overwhelms the ability of the regulatory hormones or the renal system to eliminate excess calcium ions.

Hypercapnic respiratory failure: A failure in ventilation from an inability to expel a sufficient amount of carbon dioxide.

Hyperchloremia: An electrolyte disorder in which there is an excess amount of chloride in the blood.

Hyperglycemic hyperosmolar nonketotic syndrome: A medical emergency primarily affecting patients with type 2 diabetes manifested by a blood sugar > 600 mg/dL and plasma osmolality of 310 mOsm/L.

Hyperkalemia: Results when potassium accumulates in the *extracellular* fluid to a level greater than 5.3 mEq/L.

Hypermagnesemia: An increased intake or decreased excretion of magnesium in the extracellular compartment.

Hypernatremia: A serum sodium level > 147 mEq/L.

Hyperosmolality: Depletion of the plasma volume, a serum osmolality > 295 mOsm/kg.

Hyperosmolar fluid volume deficit: Fluid deficit that occurs when more fluid is lost than sodium.

Hypervolemia: An overabundance of fluid in the intravascular compartment.

Hypervolemic hyponatremia: The result of an increase in both water and sodium, with a more significant water gain.

Hypoalbuminemia: Low serum protein.

Hypocalcemia: A lack of ingestion or absorption of the mineral calcium.

Hypochloremia: Low serum chloride level < 98 mEq/L.

Hypodipsia: A loss of the ability to sense thirst.

Hypokalemia: A serum level of potassium below 3.5 mEq/L.

Hypomagnesemia: A condition that results from decreased intake or absorption of magnesium or excessive loss.

Hyponatremia: A serum sodium < 135 mEq/L.

Hypoosmolality: A serum osmolality < 280 mOsm/kg.

Hypoventilation: Caused by a variety of conditions that results in decreased pO_2 and increased pCO_2 levels.

Hypovolemic hyponatremia: A dramatic decrease in extracellular fluid volume leading to excessive sodium loss.

Hypovolemic shock: A shock state occurring when 15–20% of the intravascular blood volume is lost.

Interstitial fluid: Fluid between or surrounding the cell.

Interstitial fluid osmotic (oncotic) pressure: The force supplied by particles in the interstitial fluid that pull fluid into the interstitial area.

Intracellular fluid: Fluid within the body cell.

Intrapulmonary shunt: Occurs when blood passes by alveoli that are filled with fluid and cannot participate with gas exchange.

Intravascular fluid: Fluid inside the vascular system.

Isoosmolar fluid volume deficit: Fluid deficit that occurs when sodium and water are lost in equal amounts.

Isotonic fluid volume excess: Fluid overload that results from a decreased elimination of sodium and water.

Kussmaul respirations: A breathing pattern of deep rapid respirations.

Left-sided cardiac failure: When the heart can no longer pump a sufficient amount of blood to supply the tissues, causing blood to back up into the left atrium and pulmonary veins.

Left ventricular ejection fraction: The amount of blood ejected from the heart per beat taking into consideration the entire amount of blood available per beat.

Magnesium: The second most prevalent cation in the intracellular fluid.

Neurogenic shock: A shock state that occurs secondary to a loss of vasomotor tone resulting in vasodilation.

Obstructive shock: A shock state that occurs secondary to a mechanical obstruction interrupting blood flow through the circulation, heart, or lungs.

Orthopnea: Shortness of breath in a recumbent position.

Osmolality: The osmolar concentration in 1 kilogram of water; used most often when referring to fluids inside the body.

Osmolarity: The osmolar concentration of 1 liter of solution; used most often when referring to solutions and fluids outside the body.

Osmoreceptors: Sensory neurons located on or near the thirst center of the hypothalamus that decrease or expand in size according to an increase or decrease in extracellular osmolality.

Osmosis: The distribution of water from a lesser area of solute concentration to a higher area of solute concentration.

Paroxysmal nocturnal dyspnea: Sudden intermittent spasms of difficult breathing occurring at night.

Passive transport: The passive movement of molecules dependent on the osmolarity of a solution involving movement from areas of greater to lesser concentration.

Phospholipids: Fat-containing molecules of phosphate that help form the cell membrane.

Poikilothermia: A temperature dysfunction resulting in the body taking on the temperature of the environment.

Potassium: The primary intracellular cation, assuming the role of sodium inside the cells and regulating intracellular osmolality.

Primary active transport: A transporter that uses an initial source of energy to carry a substance.

Proteins: A major component of the cell membrane that acts as carriers to pass compounds or channels to exchange electrolytes through the cell membrane.

Pulmonary edema: When the alveoli of the lungs fill with serosanguineous fluid.

Pulse pressure: An indicator of stroke volume, measured as the difference between the systolic and diastolic pressures.

Secondary active transport: A transporter that uses energy obtained from primary active transport.

Second-degree burn: Involves a partial thickness injury to the tissue, destroying the epidermis and damaging the dermis. Second-degree burns are classified as superficial or deep.

Septic shock: A shock state that occurs secondary to microorganisms entering the bloodstream.

Shock: A syndrome of life-threatening hemodynamic imbalance leading to poor perfusion and an inadequate supply of oxygen and nutrients to the cells.

Sodium: The most important cation in the extracellular fluid.

Sodium potassium pump: A form of active transport present in all cells to keep potassium levels high and sodium levels low inside the cell and potassium levels low and sodium levels high outside the cell.

Syndrome of inappropriate antidiuretic hormone: Occurs when the feedback loop for the release and inhibition of antidiuretic hormone malfunctions, allowing antidiuretic hormone to be continuously secreted, resulting in clinical manifestations of water intoxication.

Systolic failure: Occurs when the left ventricle (systolic function) is affected by an event that affects the contractility of the cardiac muscle fibers, making the left ventricle unable to pump the blood effectively and empty completely.

Third-degree burn: A full thickness burn that destroys the epidermis, dermis, and epidermal appendages.

Transcellular fluid compartment: The third fluid compartment of the body that includes fluid located in the peritoneal, pleural, and pericardial cavities; cerebrospinal fluid; and fluid within the joint spaces and gastrointestinal tract.

Trousseau's sign: A carpal spasm that results from local ulnar and median nerve ischemia when a blood pressure cuff is inflated on the upper arm above the systolic pressure.

Tubular reabsorption: The movement of a substance from the filtrate of the tubular lumen into the peritubular capillaries.

Tubular secretion: Movement of a substance from the peritubular capillaries into the lumen of the tubule.

Ventilation-perfusion (V/Q) mismatch: An imbalance between alveolar ventilation and pulmonary capillary blood flow.

INDEX

pH 7.35 - 7.45

PCO$_2$ 45 - 35